OXFORD MEDICAL PUBLICATIONS

*Regional Anaesthesia in Babies and Children*

# Regional Anaesthesia in Babies and Children

*J. M. Peutrell and S. J. Mather*

OXFORD   NEW YORK   MELBOURNE
OXFORD UNIVERSITY PRESS
1997

Oxford University Press, Great Clarendon Street, Oxford OX2 6DP

Oxford   New York

Athens   Auckland   Bangkok   Bogota   Bombay   Buenos Aires
Calcutta   Cape Town   Dar es Salaam   Delhi   Florence   Hong Kong
Istanbul   Karachi   Kuala Lumpur   Madras   Madrid   Melbourne
Mexico City   Nairobi   Paris   Singapore   Taipei   Tokyo   Toronto

and associated companies in
Berlin   Ibadan

Oxford is a trade mark of Oxford University Press

Published in the United States
by Oxford University Press Inc., New York

A catalogue record for this book is available from the British Library

Library of Congress Cataloging in Publication Data
Peutrell, J. M. (Jane M.)
Regional anaesthesia in babies and children / J. M. Peutrell and S. J. Mather.
(Oxford medical publications)
Includes bibliographical references and index.
1. Conduction anesthesia in children.   I. Mather, S. James.   II. Title.
III. Series.
[DNLM: 1. Anesthesia, Conduction–in infancy & childhood.
2. Anesthesia, Conduction–methods.   WO 300 P514r   1996]
RD84.P48   1996     617.9′64′083–dc20       95–43194
ISBN 0 19 262425 3 (Hbk)    ISBN 0 19 262424 5 (Pbk)

Typeset by EXPO Holdings, Malaysia

Printed in Great Britain by
Bookcraft (Bath) Ltd,
Midsomer Norton, Avon.

# Preface

This book is a practical manual designed to remind those who have been taught, and to assist in the teaching of those learning, the techniques of regional anaesthesia in babies and children. It is not intended as a substitute for direct training from experts and we do not recommend anaesthetists teach themselves the techniques.

Regional anaesthesia is currently undergoing a renaissance in paediatric anaesthetic practice, particularly in day-case surgery, for post-operative pain relief, and in ex-premature babies. Light general anaesthesia combined with an appropriate nerve block fulfils many of the requirements of an ideal anaesthetic for day-case surgery in children: rapid emergence with prolonged post-operative pain relief. Subarachnoid or caudal blocks are used in some specialist centres in awake ex-premature babies to try to reduce the incidence of post-operative apnoea after simple operations such as inguinal herniotomy. The importance of good post-operative pain relief after major surgery is now acknowledged, and infusions through catheters of local anaesthetics and other drugs are used increasingly to continue regional analgesia post-operatively.

The two introductory chapters of this book describe the relevant differences of pharmacology and the general practical aspects of regional anaesthesia. The book is then divided into sections describing the nerve blocks of the major anatomical regions of the body. The descriptions of the different blocks can be read independently and include the relevant anatomy, indications, specific contraindications, equipment, drugs and dosages. The descriptions conclude with a step-by-step guide to each block illustrated by photographs and diagrams. References are not usually cited within the text but are given, along with any suggested further reading, at the end of each description.

We hope this is a book anaesthetists will find useful in their daily clinical practice and that it will be kept in the anaesthetic room and not in the library.

*Plymouth*          J. M. P.
*Bristol*           S. J. M.
August 1996

# *Acknowledgements*

The authors are particularly indebted to Ian Ball for writing an excellent chapter on local anaesthesia in paediatric dentistry and also to the Department of Medical Illustration, Bristol Royal Infirmary for producing the photographs and drawings. We would also like to thank Ian Kestin for his encouragement and critical reviewing, David Hughes for demonstrating some of the arm blocks, and the children who volunteered to be our models.

Several illustrations are reproduced with kind permission of the authors and/or publishers and thanks are due to *Anaesthesia Intensive Care*, *Regional Anaesthesia*, Mac Keith Press and *Developmental Medicine and Child Neurology*, *Paediatric Anaesthesia*, and Elsevier Science, The Netherlands.

Finally, we must record our gratitude to our long-suffering secretaries Ann Bassett and Jane McLean for their untiring help in preparing the manuscript.

# Contents

# Part 1
## Background and principles of regional anaesthesia in children

# 1

# *General aspects of regional anaesthesia in children and babies*

## J. M. PEUTRELL

### INTRODUCTION

Regional techniques are usually combined with light general anaesthesia in children. Regional blocks provide prolonged and reasonably predictable postoperative pain relief which is particularly advantageous for children having day-case surgery. Additional analgesia (e.g. non-steroidal anti-inflammatory drugs or paracetamol) can be given to obtain adequate blood concentrations before the block has worn off. Techniques using local anaesthetics provide analgesia without the side-effects of opioids (e.g. nausea, vomiting, sedation, and ventilatory depression). The concomitant motor block is sometimes useful to immobilize limbs after operations on nerves or tendons.

Regional anaesthesia is occasionally used in awake children, for example:

(1)  as a safe alternative to general anaesthesia in older children at risk of malignant hyperpyrexia (e.g. for muscle biopsy);
(2)  to provide pain relief after trauma (e.g. femoral nerve block for a fractured shaft of femur);
(3)  for suturing small lacerations;
(4)  for minor dental surgery;
(5)  for some operations in older, co-operative children (e.g. brachial plexus block for operations on the hand);
(6)  to separate preputial adhesions after application of topical anaesthetics;
(7)  to try and reduce the incidence of postoperative apnoea in ex-premature babies (e.g. subarachnoid or caudal blocks for inguinal herniotomy or cystoscopy).

Most problems, side-effects, and complications found in adults can occur in children, but particular difficulties are:

### Lack of sedation

Regional blocks with local anaesthetics provide analgesia without sedation. Absence of sedation despite an adequate sensory block may make some young children difficult to nurse if local anaesthetic techniques alone are used for postoperative pain relief.

### Greater potential for toxic side-effects

The potential for local anaesthetic toxicity is higher in babies because the blood concentrations of binding proteins (principally alpha$_1$ acid glycoprotein) are reduced, increasing the free fraction of local anaesthetic.

## GENERAL FACILITIES FOR REGIONAL ANAESTHESIA

Regional anaesthetic techniques have two serious and immediate complications:

(1) intravascular injection of local anaesthetic producing toxic effects on the central nervous and cardiovascular systems;
(2) subarachnoid injection of large doses of local anaesthetic during extradural or interscalene blocks.

Regional anaesthetic techniques should be only used if there are facilities to manage these complications. Except for awake children having minor blocks with small doses of local anaesthetics, the following are needed:

(1) adequate monitoring: electrocardiograph, non-invasive blood pressure, and pulse oximetry;
(2) a well-trained assistant able to maintain a child's airway and interpret monitoring;
(3) secure intravenous access;
(4) resuscitation equipment and drugs to treat the effects of local anaesthetic toxicity or a total spinal block.

## ASEPTIC TECHNIQUE

Equipment must be sterile. The anaesthetist should wear sterile gloves for all procedures and a full aseptic technique should be used for all central blocks or if catheters are left in place.

### Skin cleansing

The microbes found on healthy skin are not usually pathogenic, although *Staphylococcus aureus* can colonize the nostrils, axillae, and perineum of healthy people. Pathogens are found on diseased skin (e.g. psoriasis and eczema). Twenty-fifty per cent of all skin microbes lie in follicles or crevices or are protected by lipids or squames.

The skin should be disinfected because infection is potentially such a serious complication of regional anaesthesia. An antiseptic solution containing alcohol is recommended (e.g. chlorhexidine in 70 per cent ethyl alcohol or povidone-iodine in alcohol). Friction is important when applying antiseptic solutions to disrupt the protective squames and lipids. Solutions should be allowed to dry to give them time time to work and to reduce the risk of introducing potentially neurotoxic agents on to nerves. About 80 per cent of skin bacteria are killed if 0.5 per cent chlorhexidine in 70 per cent alcohol is rubbed on the skin and allowed to dry for 30 seconds.

### FURTHER READING

Preparing the skin for injections and venepuncture. *Drug and Therapeutics Bulletin* (1972), **10**, 73–5.

Lewis, M. J. (1975). Skin preparation before injection. *Nursing Times*, **71**, 786–7.

### NEEDLES

Nerves can be damaged by needles, neurotoxic components of local anaesthetic solutions, and ischaemia caused by pressure from intraneural injection. A variety of needle tips have been designed in an attempt to reduce neural damage but the comparative risks of each are not known. In animal models long-bevelled needles are more likely to impale a nerve than short-bevelled needles, but short-bevelled needles cause more severe and longer-lasting injuries after an intraneural injection. There is greater nerve disruption if a long-bevelled needle is introduced with its bevel at right angles to the nerve fibres. There is no evidence that the incidence of neuropathy is increased by seeking paraesthesia or decreased by using a nerve stimulator.

Shorter-bevelled needles are advantageous in children, in whom fascial planes are much thinner, because it is easier to appreciate the changes in tissue resistance and 'fascial clicks' are more distinct.

Short needles are stiffer and easier to control in infants and small children.

### Needles for peripheral nerve blocks

A 2.5 cm (1 inch) needle with a short bevel is suitable for most peripheral nerve blocks (Fig. 1.1) and allows a sensitive appreciation of changes in tissue resistance. The Plexufix® (B. Braun Med. Ltd) has a 45° bevel and an extension tube to connect the needle with the syringe. The operator can hold the needle still while an assistant injects local anaesthetic (an 'immobile needle' technique).

A 25 g hypodermic or peribulbar block needle can be used for subcutaneous infiltration of nerves (e.g. radial, saphenous and superficial peroneal nerves, ring infiltration of penis). Longer needles with short bevels (e.g. 2 inch (50 mm) Plexufix®, lumbar puncture needles, or 50 mm insulated needles) are useful for sciatic nerve block in larger children.

### Needles for brachial plexus blocks

Several kits have been developed for brachial plexus block. Examples include the brachial plexus set manufactured by Arrow® and the Contiplex® brachial plexus kit manufactured by B. Braun Med Ltd (Fig. 1.2).

The brachial plexus set (Arrow®) has a catheter and an 18 g cannula over a 20 g needle with a bullet-shaped tip and lateral distal eye. The bullet-shaped tip is designed to reduce nerve damage (Fig. 1.3). The Contiplex® brachial plexus kit (B. Braun Med Ltd) comprises a cannula over a 30° short-bevelled needle (Fig. 1.3) and a radiopaque polyamide catheter.

The Arrow® International Inc needle can be used as an insulated needle. The cannula is advanced when the plexus has been

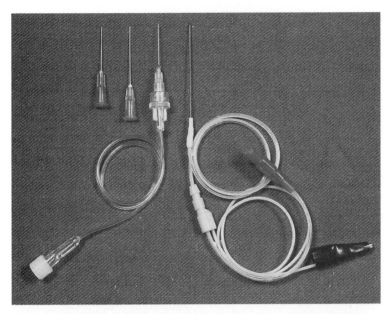

**Fig. 1.1**  From left to right: 25 g, 2.5 cm hypodermic needle used for subcutaneous infiltration (Microlance® Becton & Dickinson UK Ltd); a 25 g, 3 cm peribulbar block needle (Osborn & Simmons); an uninsulated, 25 g, 2.5 cm short-bevelled needle with an extension tube for use with an immobile needle technique (Plexufix®, B. Braun Med Ltd); an insulated, 5 cm, 22 g needle with a crocodile clip to connect to a peripheral nerve stimulator and extension tube (Vygon UK Ltd).

identified. Catheters can then be threaded, left in place and used to inject or infuse local anaesthetic solutions.

**Needles for lumbar puncture**

A lumbar puncture needle (Fig. 1.4) should have:

(1)  a stylet to reduce the risk of implantation dermoid;
(2)  a short bevel so that:
    (a)  changes in tissue resistance are easily appreciated,
    (b)  the bevel is less likely to straddle the dura, leading to incomplete injection of local anaesthetic into the subarachnoid space,
    (c)  bone and cartilage are less easily penetrated;

(3)  a short length so that the needle is easy to handle in small
     children;
(4)  a clear hub so that cerebrospinal fluid is clearly seen.

Three types of needle are used for subarachnoid anaesthesia:

(1)  cutting (Quincke and diamond-point);
(2)  short-bevelled;
(3)  atraumatic (Whitacre and Sprotte).

### *Spinal needles with cutting bevels*

Lumbar puncture needles with cutting tips usually have primary
and secondary bevels. The orientation of the secondary to the
primary bevel is 90° in the diamond point and about 30° in the
Quincke needle. The Quincke needle has a medium-length cutting
bevel. Spinocan® (B. Braun Med Ltd) and Terumo Europe

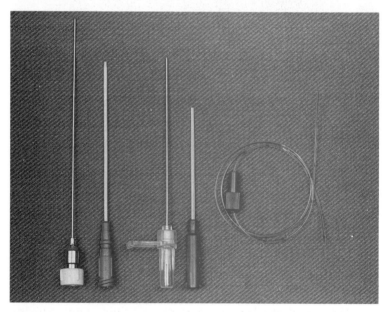

**Fig. 1.2**  Equipment for brachial plexus block: (left) the bullet-shaped
needle tip and cannula manufactured by Arrow® International, Inc.
(centre) the short-bevelled needle and cannula (Contiplex®)
manufactured by B. Braun Med Ltd, and (right) a catheter can be
threaded through both cannulae.

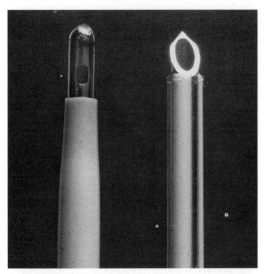

**Fig. 1.3** Needles for brachial plexus block: (left) the bullet-shaped needle tip manufactured by Arrow® International, Inc. and (right) the short-bevelled needle and cannula (Contiplex®) manufactured by B. Braun Med UK.

NV® lumbar puncture needles have modified Quincke tips with triple facet bevels. These are claimed to reduce trauma.

### Spinal needles with shorter bevels

The shorter-bevelled needles have a single straight bevel, e.g. the neonatal lumbar puncture needle manufactured by Braun®.

### Spinal needles with atraumatic tips

The designs of atraumatic lumbar puncture needles (Sprotte and Whitacre) are based on the work of Greene in the 1920s. Greene concluded that:

(1) the size of any leak of cerebrospinal fluid varied with the calibre of needle;

(2) a needle with a tapered point produced less trauma to the dura than one of the same calibre but with a blunter cutting edge.

*J. M. Peutrell*

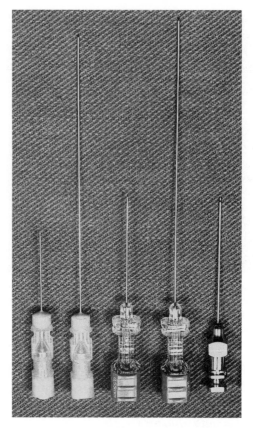

**Fig. 1.4** Needles for subarachnoid block. From left to right: 2.5 cm neonatal lumbar puncture needle (Becton Dickinson UK Ltd); 9 cm Whitacre (Becton Dickinson UK Ltd); 3.5 cm Sprotte (Pajunk®); 9 cm Sprotte (Pajunk®); 4 cm Howard Jones (Pharma-plast Ltd, Steriseal Division).

Post-lumbar puncture headache (PLPH) is thought to result from a leak of cerebrospinal fluid. The incidence of PLPH in adults is reduced by atraumatic needles.

Two types of atraumatic spinal needles are in common use (Figs 1.4 and 1.5):

(1)  The Whitacre needle has a non-cutting tip shaped like the point of a pencil. The orifice lies on the shaft of the needle just proximal to the pencil point. The length of the orifice is 0.6 mm which is less than the internal diameter of the needle.

(2) The Sprotte needle has a ogival tip. The lateral orifice on the 24 g needle is 1.2 mm long and starts about 2 mm from the tip of the needle. The orifice is longer than the internal diameter of the needle and larger than in a Whitacre needle.

Several variants of these designs are available.

### Lumbar puncture needles for babies

The depth of the subarachnoid space from the skin is approximately 0.7 cm in premature and 1 cm in full-term babies. Needles should be of a short length so they are easy to handle and have a short bevel to reduce the risk of the bevel straddling the dura and to increase its sensitivity.

The 25 g 2.5 cm neonatal lumbar puncture needle manufactured by B. Braun Med Ltd is ideal. It has a short bevel, a stylet, a clear hub and a needle dead-space of 0.05 ml.

Atraumatic needles have design features making them unsuitable for use in babies (see below).

### Lumbar puncture needles in older children

The incidence of PLPH is low but increases with age. Attempts should be made to reduce the incidence in older children by using needles of small bore with atraumatic tips (Sprotte or Whitacre).

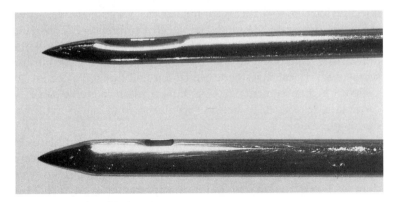

**Fig. 1.5**   The tips of a Sprotte needle (Pajunk®) (top) showing the relatively long side aperture and the ogival tip, and (bottom) the Whiteacre needle (Becton Dickinson UK Ltd) showing the smaller side aperture and the pencil-point tip.

The available atraumatic needles are not ideal. A 24 g 3.5 cm Sprotte needle is manufactured but has the disadvantage of a long lateral orifice some distance from the tip of the needle. The orifice could easily straddle the dura increasing the risk that only part of the volume of the local anaesthetic will be injected into the subarachnoid space. The lateral aperture of the Whitacre needle is much shorter and is less likely to straddle the dura. Only 9 cm needles are manufactured and these are difficult to manipulate in small children.

## Needles for extradural block

### Caudal extradural needles

A caudal needle with a short bevel has several advantages compared with standard cutting needles:

(1) a 'pop' is usually felt as the sacro-coccygeal membrane is perforated;
(2) there is a lower incidence of penetrating blood vessels, bone, and cartilage.

The needle should also have a stylet to reduce the risk of implantation dermoid. Shorter-bevelled lumbar puncture needles (20 or 22 g) are ideal. Alternatively, 18 or 20 g intravenous cannulae can be used. Although these do not have solid obturators, the metal needles are removed along with any core of tissue before injecting local anaesthetic. A cannula gives a very positive feel as its shoulders penetrate the sacro-coccygeal membrane. The cannula can then be advanced 1–2 cm over the needle and the needle withdrawn. If it cannot be advanced easily, it does not lie within the sacral canal. Local anaesthetic can be injected through a cannula at a slightly higher segmental level and, particularly in awake babies, a cannula is less likely to become displaced from the sacral canal during injection.

Extradural catheters can be threaded from the sacral hiatus in babies and young children. A baby has a relatively flat sacrum (see Fig. 12.8) and a cannula with an end-hole may be more likely than a Tuohy needle to guide a catheter cranially. A 23 g extradural catheter threads through a 20 g intravenous cannula. An 18 or 19 g Tuohy needle can be used to site extradural catheters from the sacral hiatus in older children.

### Needles for lumbar and thoracic extradural block

Lumbar and thoracic extradural catheters are usually threaded through Tuohy needles. The Tuohy needle has a rounded tip and a distal side aperture (Fig. 1.6). The tip is designed to reduce the incidence of dural puncture and vascular trauma and guide the catheter along the neuroaxis.

Needles and catheters are available in a variety of lengths and gauges according to the weight of the child (see Table 12.2). Tuohy needles—5 cm, 19 g are manufactured for use in babies and small children (Fig. 1.7). These have a small aperture to allow placement of a catheter in a narrow extradural space and a short length, making them easier to control in small children. Adult needles (8 or 9 cm long and 17 or 18 g) are used in older children.

## FURTHER READING

Chambers, W. A. (1992). Peripheral nerve damage and regional anaesthesia. *British Journal of Anaesthesia*, **69**, 429–30.

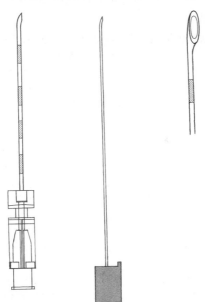

**Fig. 1.6** The 5 cm Tuohy needle for extradural anaesthesia in children (Portex Ltd) (*left*), its obturator (*centre*), and details showing the rounded tip with a distal side aperture (*right*).

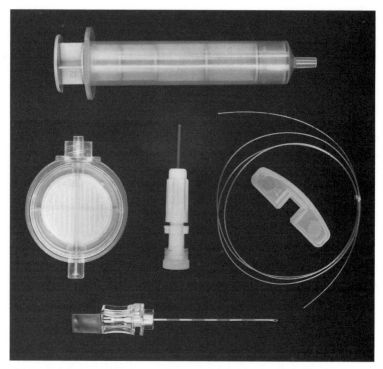

**Fig. 1.7** The paediatric extradural kit manufactured by Portex Ltd containing a 19 g, 5 cm Tuohy needle and attachable wings, a 23 g catheter, a loss of resistance syringe, a 0.22 $\mu$m bacterial filter, and a connector.

Dixon, C. L. (1991). The Sprotte, Whitacre, and Quincke spinal needles. *Anesthesiology Review*, **18**, 42–7.

Moore, D. C., Mulroy, M. F., and Thompson, G. E. (1994). Peripheral nerve damage and regional anaesthesia. *British Journal of Anaesthesia*, **73**, 435–6.

Sethna, N. F. and Berde, C. B. (1992). Pediatric regional anesthesia equipment. *International Anesthesiology Clinics*, **30**, 163–76.

## REFERENCES

Rice, A. S. C., and McMahon, S. B. (1992). Peripheral nerve injury caused by injection needles used in regional anaesthesia: influence of bevel configuration, studied in a rat model. *British Journal of Anaesthesia*, **69**, 433–8.

Selander, D., Dhunér, K.-G., and Lundberg, G. (1977). Peripheral nerve injury due to injection needles used for regional anaesthesia. *Acta Anaesthesiologica Scandinavica*, **21**, 182–8.

## LOCAL ANAESTHETIC SOLUTIONS

Local anaesthetic solutions in clinically useful concentrations are not neurotoxic if applied to the outside of an intact nerve. Intrafascicular injections produce axonal degeneration and damage to the blood–nerve barrier. The degree of damage caused by an intrafascicular injection of bupivacaine is not different from that seen after injection of saline. Adrenaline increases the damage, probably by causing vasoconstriction of neural blood vessels.

Sodium bisulphite and related compounds are added as antioxidants to some solutions of local anaesthetics, particularly those containing adrenaline. Sodium bisulphite can cause irreversible nerve damage and the risk is increased if large volumes at a low pH are used. Local anaesthetic solutions free of preservatives should be used for regional anaesthesia to reduce the risk of nerve damage. Adrenaline can be added to solutions immediately before use.

## FURTHER READING

Chambers, W. A. (1992). Peripheral nerve damage and regional anaesthesia. *British Journal of Anaesthesia*, **69**, 429–30.

## REFERENCES

Selander, D., Brattsand, R., Lundborg, G., Nordborg, C., and Olsson, Y. (1979). Local anesthetics: importance of mode of application, concentration and adrenaline for the appearance of nerve lesions. *Acta Anaesthesiologica Scandinavica*, **23**, 127–36.

Wang, B. C., Hillman, D. E., Spielholz, N. I., and Turndorf, H. (1984). Chronic neurological deficits and nesacaine-CE – an effect of the anesthetic, 2-chloroprocaine, or the antioxidant, sodium bisulfite? *Anesthesia Analgesia*, **63**, 445–7.

## PARTICULATE FILTERS

Infusions of local anaesthetics should be filtered using 0.22 $\mu$m filters to exclude bacteria and glass particles. The filter aspiration needle manufactured by Monoject® has a 5 μm stainless steel filter designed to exclude particles of glass and it is used to draw local anaesthetic solutions from glass ampoules.


## PERIPHERAL NERVE STIMULATORS

Nerves are located more accurately in children using a peripheral nerve stimulator because the anatomy is variable and para-esthesiae cannot be elicited in anaesthetized children. Precise location reduces the amount of local anaesthetic needed to successfully block nerve transmission.


### Electrophysiology of peripheral nerve stimulators

A threshold stimulus must be applied to a nerve for a minimum length of time to propagate a nerve impulse. A smaller current must be applied for a longer time than a larger current to generate a nerve impulse. The rheobase is the minimum current that will generate a nerve impulse (Fig. 1.8).

The chronaxie is the duration of stimulus that just generates a nerve impulse at twice the rheobase. Larger myelinated nerve fibres have smaller chronaxies than smaller non-myelinated nerves, which means that motor fibres (A alpha) can be stimulated without stimulating pain fibres (A delta and C fibres). Mixed nerves can therefore be found in awake patients by eliciting a twitch response without causing pain.


### Ideal characteristics of a peripheral nerve stimulator

The ideal characteristics of a peripheral nerve stimulator are given in Table 1.1. A nerve stimulator usually has a variable voltage. The current output varies directly with the voltage and indirectly with the external resistance (e.g. body tissues, connectors, needles) and the internal resistance of the nerve stimulator, i.e.

$$\text{current} = \frac{\text{voltage}}{\text{resistance}} \text{ (Ohm's law)}.$$

The resistances of body tissues, connectors and needles can vary twentyfold. The internal resistance of the nerve stimulator must

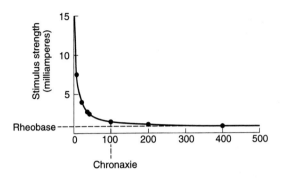

Fig. 1.8 Strength duration curve of a cat sciatic nerve, showing the rheobase (the smallest current that stimulates the nerve when applied for a long time) and the chronaxie (the duration of stimulus applied at twice the rheobase that just generates a nerve impulse). (From Figure 1 in Pither, C. E., Raj, R. P., and Ford, D. J. (1986). The use of peripheral nerve stimulators for regional anesthesia. A review of experimental characteristics, technique, and critical applications. *Regional Anesthesia*, **10**, 49–58 with kind permission.)

be large enough to provide a constant current output at a given voltage. The current output should be variable but alter linearly with changes of the control dial and range from 0.1 to 10 mA. The current delivered should be displayed accurately on a digital meter: a low current output will stimulate a nerve when the needle lies immediately adjacent to whereas a higher output is needed if the needle lies several centimetres away. The polarity of the leads must be marked clearly; the cathode is the negative lead and the anode is the positive lead. The negative output is usually coloured black but this varies with manufacturer. Four times more current is needed to depolarize a nerve if the needle is attached to the anode than if attached to the cathode. The duration of the pulse of current should be short (50–100 μseconds) because a short pulse is a better discriminator of the distance between the needle and nerve. The nerve stimulator should be able to deliver repeated current pulses at a frequency of 1 second⁻¹.

The peripheral nerve stimulator manufactured by Bard Critical Care (Fig. 1.9) has high and low current outputs and is designed for monitoring of neuromuscular function and locating mixed

**Table 1.1** Desirable characteristics of a peripheral nerve stimulator (Pither *et al.* 1986)

Constant current output
Clear meter reading to 0.1 mA (preferably digital)
Variable output control
Linear output
Clearly marked polarity
Short pulse width
Pulse of 1 Hz
Battery indicator
High and low output
High-quality clips (e.g. crocodile clips)

peripheral nerves. The low output is used during regional anaesthesia.

## Needles for use with peripheral nerve stimulators

Insulated and uninsulated needles can be used with peripheral nerve stimulators but they have different patterns of current density; this affects their use in clinical practice. The advantages and disadvantages of insulated and un-insulated needles are summarized in Table 1.2.

### Insulated needles

The pattern of current density is a sphere around the tip of an insulated needle (Fig. 1.10a) with the highest density at the tip of the needle. The current needed to stimulate a nerve is lowest when the needle tip lies adjacent to the nerve. The current needed to generate a nerve impulse rises rapidly as the needle is advanced beyond the nerve. The needle tip lies virtually adjacent to the nerve if a muscle twitch is elicited by a stimulus of 0.3–0.5 mA.

### Uninsulated needles

The maximum current density around an uninsulated needle is just proximal to the tip of the needle, but significant current extends along the length of the needle (Fig. 1.10b). Only about 30 per cent of the current is concentrated at the needle tip. The current needed to stimulate a nerve is lowest when the tip of the

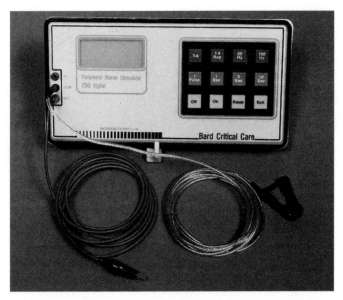

**Fig. 1.9** The peripheral nerve stimulator manufactured by Bard Critical Care can be used to locate mixed peripheral nerves and monitor neuromuscular function. It has low and high current outputs and a digital display.

**Table 1.2** Summary of differences between insulated and uninsulated needles (Pither *et al.* 1986)

| Insulated | Uninsulated |
|---|---|
| Greater accuracy | Accurate |
| Expensive | Very cheap |
| Often unobtainable | Readily available |
| No stimulation from shaft | Local stimulation from shaft |
| Less current required | Slightly more current required |
| Minimum current on nerve | Minimum current just past nerve |
| Can alter feel of tissues | No alteration in feel of tissues |

needle lies just beyond the nerve but will remain low as the needle is advanced because of stimulation from the needle shaft. In practice, a higher current (e.g. 0.5–1.0 mA for the femoral nerve and 1–2 mA for the sciatic nerve) is needed to stimulate nerves using

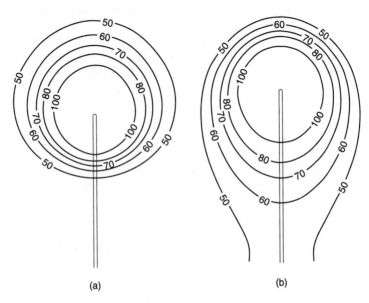

**Fig. 1.10**   The pattern of current density around (a) insulated and
(b) uninsulated needles (relative scale). (Based on Figure based on
Figures 2 and 3 in Bashein, G. *et al.* (1984). Electrical nerve location.
Numerical and electrophoretic comparisons of insulated versus
uninsulated needles. *Anesthesia Analgesia*, **63**, 919–24, with kind
permission.)

non-insulated needles. The needle should be withdrawn from its
position of maximum stimulation until a motor response is just
elicited. Loss of muscle twitch after the injection of 1–2 ml of
local anaesthetic strongly suggests that the needle tip is
immediately adjacent to the nerve.

### Reference electrodes

The reference electrode (e.g. an electrocardiograph lead) should
be applied to dry skin avoiding the course of superficial nerves.

### Using a peripheral nerve stimulator

1. The anode (positive lead) is attached to the reference electrode.
2. The needle is advanced a short distance through the skin over
   the course of the nerve and then connected to the cathode (negative lead) with crocodile clips. The negative jack of the nerve
   stimulator is usually black but does vary with manufacturer.

3. The nerve stimulator is adjusted to deliver a current output of 5–10 mA. This may produce a localized muscle twitch.
4. The needle is advanced towards the nerve. A current output of 5–10 mA should stimulate the appropriate muscle groups when the needle tip is 1–2 cm from the nerve. The power of the muscle twitch increases as the needle nears the nerve. If the twitch decreases, it is probable that the needle is moving to one side of the nerve and the needle should be redirected.
5. The current output should be reduced as the needle is advanced. The needle lies very close to nerve when a current output of 0.1–0.5 mA through an insulated needle, or 0.5–2 mA through a non-insulated needle, produces a twitch in the appropriate muscle group.
6. An injection of 1–2 ml of local anaesthetic reduces or abolishes muscle twitching if the needle tip is very close to the nerve, by physically displacing the nerve from the needle tip. This sign is not always reliable because it can also occur when the tip of the needle lies just beyond the nerve. If the test injection does not considerably reduce the power of the muscle contraction, the needle should be removed and redirected until twitching again occurs with low current outputs. The test injection should then be repeated before the full dose of local anaesthetic is injected.

### Locating nerves by detecting mixed nerve action potentials

With this technique a mixed nerve is stimulated distally using a bipolar surface stimulator. The mixed nerve action potential is then detected proximally using an insulated needle. The advantages of this method are:

(1) there can be no direct stimulation of muscle which could give a false positive result; and
(2) in conscious patients it avoids pain from stimulation of sensory nerves or movement of injured parts caused by muscle contractions.

### FURTHER READING

Pither, C. E., Raj, R. P., and Ford, D. J. (1986). The use of peripheral nerve stimulators for regional anesthesia. A review of experimental characteristics, technique, and critical applications. *Regional Anesthesia*, **10**, 49–58.

## REFERENCES

Bashein, G., Haschke, R. H., and Ready, L. B. (1984). Electrical nerve location. Numerical and electrophoretic comparison of insulated versus uninsulated needles. *Anesthesia Analgesia*, **63**, 919–24.

Bösenberg, A. T. (1995). Lower limb nerve blocks in children using unsheathed needles and a nerve stimulator. *Anaesthesia*, **50**, 206–10.

Wee, M. Y. K., Geeurickx, A., and Wimalaratna, S. (1992). A method to facilitate regional anaesthesia by detection of mixed nerve action potentials. *British Journal of Anaesthesia*, **69**, 411–13.

## SYSTEMIC TOXICITY OF LOCAL ANAESTHETICS

Local anaesthetics are membrane stabilizers that interrupt electrical transmission along nerves by blocking sodium channels. In high blood concentrations they will have toxic effects on other excitable membranes, e.g. the brain and heart.

The usual cause of toxicity associated with regional anaesthesia is the inadvertent injection of local anaesthetic into blood vessels. The severity of symptoms will depend on the peak concentration within the blood arriving at the heart or brain. This peak concentration is determined by several factors:

### The dose of local anaesthetic

The greater the dose, the higher the blood concentration.

### The cardiac output

The cardiac output is proportional to the volume of blood in which the local anaesthetic is initially distributed. The greater the cardiac output, the lower the peak concentration of local anaesthetic.

### The speed of injection

The slower the speed of injection, the lower the blood concentration.

### Injection into vein or artery

Injection into a vein generally produces lower concentrations in the blood arriving at the brain or heart because there is significant uptake by the lungs. Direct injection into an artery (e.g. the vertebral artery during an interscalene block), retrograde flow into the cerebral circulation from an artery in the head or neck (e.g. during a mandibular nerve block), or intravenous injection in children with right to left intracardiac shunts will produce neurotoxicity with very low doses of local anaesthetics. Retrograde flow into the cerebral venous and capillary circulation can also occur from injection into extradural veins because these have no valves.

The rate of uptake of local anaesthetic from tissues into the systemic circulation depends on:

### The site of injection

The rate of uptake of local anaesthetic solutions into the systemic circulation depends on the vascularity and vascular surface area at the site of injection. Blood concentrations decrease in the following order:

(1)  topical anaesthesia of airways;
(2)  intercostal nerve block;
(3)  extradural anaesthesia from the lumbar/thoracic route;
(4)  extradural anaesthesia from the caudal route;
(5)  proximal blocks of the arm (supraclavicular > axillary);
(6)  proximal blocks of the leg (sciatic and femoral);
(7)  subcutaneous infiltration.

Uptake into the arterial circulation is also increased in children with arteriovenous malformations at the site of injection.

Widely accepted safe maximum doses for lignocaine and bupivacaine are given in Table 1.3 but these will ultimately depend on the site of injection. In adults twice as much lignocaine can be injected safely into subcutaneous tissues compared with lumbar extradural anaesthesia.

**Table 1.3**  Maximum recommended doses for lignocaine and bupivacaine in children older than 4 weeks. Doses should be reduced in neonates

| | | |
|---|---|---|
| Lignocaine | (plain) | 3 mg kg$^{-1}$ |
| | (with adrenaline) | 6 mg kg$^{-1}$ |
| Bupivacaine | (extradural) | 2.5 mg kg$^{-1}$ followed by 0.5 mg kg$^{-1}$ h$^{-1}$ |

## The addition of vasoconstrictors

The reduction in peak concentrations by the addition of vasocon-strictors depends upon the site of injection and the drug. Adrenaline significantly reduces the peak concentration of ligno-caine but has much less effect on bupivacaine. The effect on lig-nocaine is much greater after subcutaneous infiltration than after intercostal, extradural, or brachial plexus block.

## The local anaesthetic

The rate of uptake of bupivacaine from the extradural space is slower compared with lignocaine.

Local anaesthetics given as continuous infusions can accumu-late in some children even when the rate of infusion does not exceed the recommended maximum rates. The hepatic extraction of bupivacaine is concentration dependent and is lower at higher blood concentrations. The rate of excretion may be reduced further by partial resection of the liver.

The risk of toxicity can be reduced by:

(1) **NEVER** exceeding the maximum recommended doses;
(2) aspirating before and during injection;
(3) injecting the local anaesthetic slowly;
(4) observing the electrocardiograph throughout the injection of local anaesthetic and stopping if there is a change in heart rate or morphology of the QRS complexes.

The use of test doses of local anaesthetics with adrenaline are discussed on p. 193.

### Neurotoxicity

Many of the signs and symptoms of local anaesthetic toxicity are masked by general anaesthesia. In a conscious patient the pattern of symptoms associated with increasing blood concentrations tend to occur in the following order, although there is variability between patients:

(1) numbness of the tongue and around the mouth;
(2) light-headedness;
(3) tinnitus;
(4) visual disturbances which may cause oscillations of the eyes;

(5)  slurring of speech;
(6)  irrational conversation;
(7)  loss of consciousness;
(8)  seizures;
(9)  apnoea.

Younger children may not complain of any of these symptoms and restlessness caused by cerebral toxicity may be misinterpreted as pain or hunger. Convulsions can occur in children with plasma concentrations of bupivacaine greater than 2 $\mu$g ml$^{-1}$. They are very unlikely with infusion rates less than 0.5 mg kg$^{-1}$ h$^{-1}$ unless there are additional risk factors, e.g. postoperative fever and a past history of febrile convulsions, epilepsy, hypomagnesaemia, hypophosphataemia, or hyponatraemia.

### Treatment of neurotoxicity
A high index of suspicion should be maintained in any child having a continuous infusion of local anaesthetic who becomes agitated, confused, or who complains of any symptoms associated with toxicity. The infusion or injection should be stopped and blood taken to measure the concentration of local anaesthetic. No further treatment is needed unless the child starts to have fits.

### Maintaining adequate oxygenation and ventilation
Acidosis and hypoxia potentiate the toxic effects of local anaesthetics. Acidosis decreases protein binding, increases the intracellular ionized fraction, increases blood flow to the brain, and delays distribution to muscle and fat. Acidosis and hypoxia probably make the heart and brain more vulnerable to the effects of local anaesthetics. A convulsing child should be given a high inspired oxygen concentration and his or her lungs should be ventilated if there is apnoea or if breathing is inadequate.

### Stopping the convulsions
Convulsions caused by intravascular injection of local anaesthetic are often short-lived and do not recur after effective treatment. They occur during the initial high blood concentrations and stop as the blood concentration falls. There may be a greater propensity for continuing convulsions if they have occurred during a continuous infusion of local anaesthetic. A convulsion should be treated if it has not stopped after 20–30 seconds, using either thiopentone 2–3 mg kg$^{-1}$ or diazemuls® 0.25–0.4 mg kg$^{-1}$.

## Cardiotoxicity

Although most of the electrophysiological effects of lignocaine and bupivacaine are similar, the two drugs have different adverse effects on the heart and brain: the ratio of lignocaine to bupivacaine that produces myocardial depression, neural blockade, and convulsions is 4 : 1, but the ratio of doses facilitating arrhythmias is 16 : 1. Hypoxia, acidosis, hyperkalaemia, and hyponatraemia potentiate the toxic effects of local anaesthetics and slow the rate of their dissociation from sodium channels.

Lignocaine is a class I antiarrhythmic drug. In toxic doses it impairs myocardial contractility and induces hypotension, bradycardia, and asystole. Lignocaine does not facilitate re-entrant ventricular tachy-arrhythmias in animal models except in extremely high doses.

Bupivacaine in toxic doses impairs myocardial contractility, causes bradycardia and hypotension, and is associated with ventricular tachy-arrhythmias that are difficult to treat. Bupivacaine has a direct effect on cardiac tissue to facilitate re-entrant arrhythmias. There may also be a neurogenic component: bupivacaine can increase the autonomic outflow by blocking GABA ($\gamma$-aminobutyric acid) receptors in the brainstem (these neurones inhibit sympathetic and parasympathetic outflow). Neurogenic-mediated ventricular arrhythmias may be controlled by GABA agonists, e.g. benzodiazepines.

The electrocardiograph changes associated with bupivacaine toxicity are:

(1) prolongation of the PR and QT intervals;
(2) a wide QRS complex;
(3) development of a U wave (a 'slow wave') after the T wave;
(4) AV block;
(5) polymorphic ventricular tachycardia;
(6) electromechanical dissociation;
(7) asystole.

Ventricular tachycardia may be associated with undulating complexes similar to those in the syndrome of torsade de pointes.

### Treatment of cardiotoxicity

The initial treatment of cardiotoxicity follows the principles of basic and advanced life support, including cardioversion

(Fig. 1.11a–c). Aggressive treatment of cardiovascular and central nervous toxicity improves survival in animals. Bupivacaine remains in cardiac tissue much longer than lignocaine and cannot be eliminated without sustained and effective cardiac massage. Local anaesthetic toxicity is potentiated by hypoxia and acidosis, and adequate oxygenation and ventilation are essential.

Recommendations for the drug treatment of ventricular arrhythmias are based on research in animals and case reports of successful resuscitation in humans.

### *Adrenaline*

Although low-dose adrenaline added to local anaesthetic solutions does not protect against bupivacaine-induced cardiac arrest, large doses are indicated to counteract the cardiovascular depressant effects of local anaesthetics. High-dose adrenaline is the mainstay of resuscitation in animal models.

### *Bretylium*

This is a class III antiarrhythmic that prolongs the effective refractory period of the action potential and inhibits re-entrant tachy-arrhythmias. Bretylium can sometimes convert ventricular tachy-arrhythmias to sinus rhythm but more commonly facilitates electrical cardioversion. The dose is 5 mg kg$^{-1}$ intravenously repeated up to 30 mg kg$^{-1}$. The antifibrillatory effects may take time to develop and resuscitation should continue for 20–30 minutes after a loading dose.

### *Phenytoin*

This is a class I$_b$ antiarrhythmic that has been used successfully in two neonates with bupivacaine toxicity to treat broad complex tachy-arrhythmias after bretylium (10 mg kg$^{-1}$) had failed to terminate the arrhythmia although cardioversion had not been attempted. The use of phenytoin for treatment of ventricular arrhythmias associated with bupivacaine has not been reported in humans elsewhere and has not been investigated in animal models. It is not recommended as first line treatment.

The initial dose is 5 mg kg$^{-1}$ injected at a rate less than or equal to 50 mg min$^{-1}$. Further doses can be given at 5 minute intervals to a maximum of 15 mg kg$^{-1}$. Phenytoin should be diluted in saline and injected into a fast-flowing intravenous infusion.

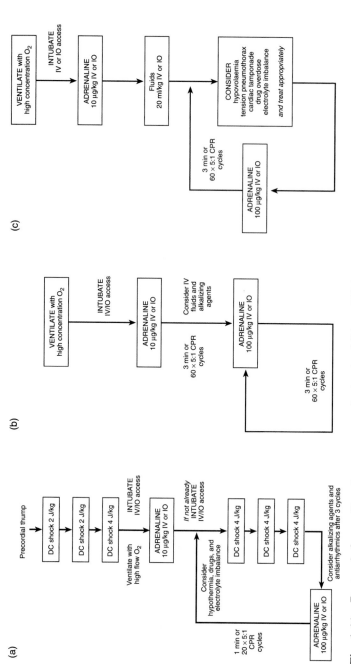

**Fig. 1.11** Protocols for cardiopulmonary resuscitation in children (IV, intravenous; IO, intra-osseous; CPR, cardiopulmonary resuscitation). (a) Ventricular fibrillation; (b) asystole; (c) electromechanical dissociation. (From the *APLS Handbook* published by the *British Medical Journal* with kind permission.)

*GABA receptor agonists (e.g. benzodiazepines)*
These may be indicated to counteract arrhythmias induced by the central nervous system effects of bupivacaine.

## FURTHER READING

Arthur, G. R. and Covino, B. G. (1991). Pharmacokinetics of local anaesthetics. *Clinical Anaesthesiology*, **5**, 635–58.

Berde, C. B. (1992). Convulsions associated with pediatric regional anesthesia. *Anesthesia Analgesia*, **75**, 164–6.

McCaughey, W. (1992). Adverse effects of local anaesthetics. *Drug Safety*, **7**, 178–89.

Reiz, S. and Nath, S. (1986). Cardiotoxicity of local anaesthetic agents. *British Journal of Anaesthesia*, **58**, 736–46.

Scott, D. B. (1986). Toxic effects of local anaesthetic agents on the central nervous system. *British Journal of Anaesthesia*, **58**, 732–5.

Scott, D. B. (1989). 'Maximum recommended doses' of local anaesthetic drugs. *British Journal of Anaesthesia*, **63**, 373–4.

Tucker, G. T. (1986). Pharmacokinetics of local anaesthetics. *British Journal of Anaesthesia*, **58**, 717–31.

## REFERENCES

Agarwal, R., Gutlove, D. P., and Lockhart, C. H. (1992). Seizures occurring in pediatric patients receiving continuous infusion of bupivacaine. *Anesthesia Analgesia*, **75**, 284–6.

Bernards, C. M., and Artru, A. A. (1991). Hexamethonium and midazolam terminate dysrhythmias and hypertension caused by intracerebroventricular bupivacaine in rabbits. *Anesthesiology*, **74**, 89–96.

Bernards, C. M., *et al.* (1989). Effect of epinephrine on central nervous system and cardiovascular system toxicity of bupivacaine in pigs. *Anesthesiology*, **71**, 711–17.

Davis, N. L., and de Jong, R. H. (1982). Successful resuscitation following massive bupivacaine overdose. *Anesthesia Analgesia*, **61**, 62–4.

de la Coussaye, J. E., Brugada, J., and Allessie, M. A. (1992). Electrophysiologic and arrhythmogenic effects of bupivacaine. *Anesthesiology*, **77**, 132–41.

Feldman, H. S., *et al.* (1991). Treatment of acute systemic toxicity after the rapid intravenous injection of bupivacaine in the conscious dog. *Anesthesia Analgesia*, **73**, 373–84.

Heavner, J. E. (1986). Cardiac dysrhythmias induced by infusion of local anaesthetics into the lateral cerebral ventricle of cats. *Anesthesia Analgesia*, **65**, 133–38.

Heavner, J. E., *et al.* (1992). Severe hypoxia enhances central nervous system and cardiovascular toxicity of bupivacaine in lightly anesthetized pigs. *Anesthesiology*, 77, 142–7.

Kasten, G. W., and Martin, S. T. (1985). Bupivacaine cardiovascular toxicity: comparison of treatment with bretylium and lidocaine. *Anesthesia Analgesia*, 64, 911–16.

Maxwell, L. G., Martin, L. D., and Yaster, M. (1994). Bupivacaine-induced cardiac toxicity in neonates: successful treatment with intravenous phenytoin. *Anesthesiology*, 80, 682–6.

Moller, R. A., and Covino, B. G. (1988). Cardiac electrophysiologic effects of lidocaine and bupivacaine. *Anesthesia Analgesia*, 67, 107–14.

Nath, S., Häggmark, S., Johansson, G., and Reiz, S. (1986). Differential depressant and electrophysiologic cardiotoxicity of local anesthetics: an experimental study with special reference to lidocaine and bupivacaine. *Anesthesia Analgesia*, 65, 1263–70.

Timour, Q., Freysz, M., Mazze, R., Couzon, P., Bertrix, L., and Faucon, G. (1990). Enhancement by hyponatremia and hyperkalemia of ventricular conduction and rhythm disorders caused by bupivacaine. *Anesthesiology*, 72, 1051–6.

Wolf, A. R., *et al.* (1993). Effect of extradural analgesia on stress responses to abdominal surgery in infants. *British Journal of Anaesthesia*, 70, 654–60.

# SYSTEMIC ANALGESICS USED TO COMPLEMENT REGIONAL ANAESTHETIC TECHNIQUES

## Children and babies older than 6 months

Single injections of local anaesthetic have a limited duration of analgesia. Systemic analgesics (e.g. paracetamol or non-steroidal anti-inflammatory drugs) should be given to ensure adequate blood concentrations before the block wears off. Analgesia obtained from continuous infusions of extradural local anaesthetics is sometimes inadequate and can be improved by the addition of non-steroidal anti-inflammatory drugs or intravenous opioids. Opioids are sedative and this may be very useful in small children. They should not be given without discussion with an anaesthetist if opioids have been injected into the subarachnoid or extradural spaces. The doses of some systemic analgesics for children aged over 6 months are given in Table 1.4.

**Table 1.4** Some systemic analgesics and their doses used to complement regional anaesthetic techniques in children and babies older than 6 months.

| | Dose | Dose interval (h) | Route |
|---|---|---|---|
| Paracetamol | 20 mg kg$^{-1}$ followed by 15 mg kg$^{-1}$ | 6 | O/R |
| Non-steroidal anti-inflammatory drugs | | | |
| diclofenac | 1 mg kg$^{-1}$ (3 mg kg$^{-1}$ 24 h$^{-1}$) | 6–8 | O/R |
| ibuprofen | 5 mg kg$^{-1}$ | 6 | O |
| Opioids | | | |
| codeine phosphate | 1–1.5 mg kg$^{-1}$ | 4 | O/IM[a] |
| dihydrocodeine | 0.5–1.0 mg kg$^{-1}$ | 4 | O |
| morphine | 50 $\mu$g kg$^{-1}$ repeated every 10 minutes until pain-free (up to 150 $\mu$g kg$^{-1}$) | 2 | IV, or loading dose followed by infusion of 10–40 $\mu$g kg$^{-1}$ h$^{-1}$ |
| pethidine | 0.5 mg kg$^{-1}$ repeated every 10 minutes until pain-free (up to 1.5 mg kg$^{-1}$) | 2 | IV, or loading dose followed by infusion of 0.1–0.4 mg kg$^{-1}$ h$^{-1}$ |

[a]cannot be given IV.    IV, intravenous; IM, intramuscular; O, oral; R, rectal.

## Babies younger than 6 months

The rate of excretion of paracetamol is not affected by age, but babies conjugate a higher proportion with sulphate rather than glucuronide compared with older children. The dose of paracetamol in babies is therefore the same as in children.

The dose of morphine should be reduced in babies younger than about 6 months because:

(1)  the rate of excretion in very young babies is reduced;
(2)  the free-fraction of drug is increased;
(3)  the disposition into the central nervous system is increased;
(4)  babies are probably more sensitive to the effects of opioids.

A loading dose of 0.05 mg $kg^{-1}$ followed by an infusion of 0.005–0.01 mg $kg^{-1}$ usually seems adequate. Babies having continuous infusions of opioids should be cared for on a high-dependency unit and monitored for apnoea and oxygen desaturation.

## REFERENCES

Bhat, R. *et al.* (1990). Pharmacokinetics of a single dose of morphine in preterm infants during the first week of life. *Journal of Pediatrics*, **117**, 477–81.

Lynn, A. M. and Slattery, J. T. (1987). Morphine pharmacokinetics in early infancy. *Anesthesiology*, **66**, 136–9.

Lynn, A. M. *et al.* (1991). Morphine partitioning between plasma and cerebrospinal fluid in monkeys. *Developmental Pharmacology and Therapeutics*, **17**, 200–4.

Miller, R. P., Roberts, R. J., and Fischer, L. J. (1976). Acetaminophen elimination kinetics in neonates, children, and adults. *Clinical Pharmacology and Therapeutics*, **19**, 284–94.

# 2
# Biology and pharmacology: some differences

S. J. MATHER

## INTRODUCTION

It is beyond the scope of this chapter to discuss the molecular basis of local anaesthetic action, which could justify a book in itself. The purpose of the following chapter is to outline some of the differences between babies and larger children and adults in the ways in which they behave toward painful stimuli and their handling of local anaesthetic drugs.

Not many years ago it was common practice to withhold analgesic drugs from babies. This attitude was based on the observation that newborn babies do not respond in the same way as older children and adults when confronted with what we would normally regard as a painful stimulus, for example a surgical incision. The further observation that babies, particularly newborns and ex-premature infants, readily stop breathing if given 'normal' therapeutic doses of opioids has led to the widespread belief that, first, neonates do not require any postoperative analgesia and, secondly, opioids are dangerous in this group. Concern is also expressed about the use of non-steroidal anti-inflammatory drugs (NSAIDs) in very young children because of possible detrimental effects on the kidney, platelet function, the gastrointestinal tract and perhaps a link with Reye's syndrome.

Undoubtedly, injudicious use of powerful respiratory depressants, including opioids, in anaesthesia may lead to potentially life-threatening apnoea.

For these reasons, and a growing concern about attenuation of the 'stress response' (Anand and Hickey 1987; McGrath and

Unnih 1987) there has been a renewed interest in local and regional analgesia in babies and children.

The use of local nerve blocks has many advantages, particularly in those children who may be sensitive to opioids or in whom sedation is undesirable. Opioids also tend to increase the time to resumption of enteral feeding and very frequently increase the incidence of vomiting, which may be as distressing as the pain being treated.

However, local anaesthetics must be used with caution. It is very easy to infiltrate a large area in a baby with the commonly used concentrations of local anaesthetic agents such that the toxic dose is exceeded. It does not look a very large volume in the syringe but it may be too much. In babies and young children one can very often reduce the concentration in order to allow a greater volume to be given and still produce a very satisfactory block. Central blocks tend to wear off more quickly in young children when compared with adults but the temptation to use higher concentrations in order to prolong the block must be resisted. If prolonged blockade is required, repeat block or an infusion is more appropriate.

Conventional methods of pain assessment, such as visual and linear analogues, which are applicable to older children, cannot be used in babies and infants. There remains the problem, then, of how to assess pain in this group. Similar responses, such as crying and tachycardia, and flexion of the limbs, can occur with both hunger and pain. Fitzgerald (1991) and her colleagues, however, maintain that a clear threshold can be seen in flexor reflex responses and this can be used as a measure of cutaneous sensory response in infants (see also Chan and Dallaire 1989). The distinction between high-threshold and low-threshold nociceptor responses is less in infants. Thresholds are apparently very low in premature infants, the flexion reflex being evoked by low-intensity stimuli such as light touch. The threshold increases with gestational age (Fig. 2.1) but even so, remains low at term (Fitzgerald *et al.* 1988). The flexion reflex, however, can be used as a measure of pain in neonates because it changes distinctly following tissue injury, the threshold for withdrawal being lower in the injured limb.

Much work on maturation of the nervous system has been done in rats, but the development of their nervous system at birth is

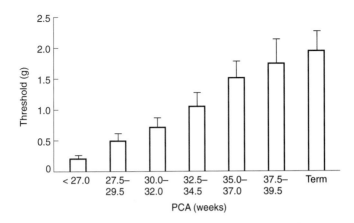

**Fig. 2.1**   Increase in threshold of flexor reflex with postconceptional age (PCA) in preterm and full-term babies. (From Fitzgerald, M., Shaw, A., and MacIntosh, N. (1988). Postnatal development of the cutaneous flexor reflex: Comparative study of preterm infants and newborn rat pups. *Developmental Medicine and Child Neurology,* **30,** 520–6; with permission.)

less complete than in humans. However, the two species can be equated (see Fig. 2.2), the first 2–3 weeks of postnatal life in the rat corresponding to 24–40 weeks' gestation in the human. It is assumed, therefore, that experiments on the rat at this stage of development can, in some measure, be extrapolated to premature and full-term human newborns.

It seems likely that from around 26 weeks' gestation human fetuses possess the anatomical infrastructure for pain pathways, although the functional basis of these connections is unknown. Neurotransmitters and their receptors undergo qualitative and quantitative development along with the anatomical maturation of the nervous system (Fitzgerald *et al.* 1991). The nervous system is certainly immature at birth, as evidenced by the 'global response' seen in newborns in response to a stimulus. This state suggests immaturity of inhibitory pathways (Ekholm 1987).

Somatosensory maturity is dependent upon many factors. C fibres grow into the cord later than A-fibres (Fitzgerald *et al.* 1987). The C-fibres also do not make connection with the substantia gelatinosa until after birth (Bicknell and Beal 1984).

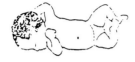  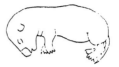

| Postmenstrual weeks | | Embryonic (E) and Postnatal (P) days |
|---|---|---|
| 5 [1] | Neural tube closes | E 10 [2] |
| 7.5 [1] | Synapses in ventral horn | E 13.5 [3] |
| 8 [1] | Afferent synapses in cord | E 14.5 [3] |
| 7.5–8 [4] | Spontaneous fetal movements | E 15 [5] |
| 7.5–8 [6] | Cutaneous reflexes (lip) | E 15 [5] |
| 9–12 [7] | SOM, SP in substantia gelatinosa | E15–17 [8] |
| 12.5 [6] | Cutaneous reflexes (foot) | E17 [5] |
| 13 [8] | Lamination in cord | E 17 [8] |
| 25 [9] | Motorneurone death complete | P0 [10] |
| 25 [8,11] | ENK in substantia gelatinosa | P1 [8] |
| 26 [12] | Thalamocortical input | P0 [13] |
| 26 [14] | Innervation of cutaneous hair follicles | P 5–7 [14] |
| 29[15] | Maturation of somatosensory evoked potential | P10 [16] |
| 30[17] | Decreased excitability of cutaneous reflexes | P14 [17] |

References:
1, Okado and Kojima (1984); 2, Altman and Bayer (1984); 3, Vaughan and Grieshaber (1973); 4, Devries *et al.* (1982); 5, Narayanan *et al.* (1971); 6, Hooker (1952); 7, Charnay *et al.* (1987); 8, Marti *et al.* (1987); 9, Forger and Breediove (1987); 10, Oppenheim (1987); 11, Charnay *et al.* (1984); 12, Mrzljak *et al.* (1988); 13, Wise and Jones (1978); 14, Fitzgerald *et al.* (1991); 15, Klimach and Cooke (1988); 16, Thairu (1971); 17, Fitzgerald *et al.* (1988).

**Fig. 2.2**   Maturation of the nervous system in humans and rats. SOM, somatostatin; SP, substance P; ENK, enkephalin. (From Fitzgerald, M. (1991). In *Proceedings of the VIth World Congress on Pain*, (ed. M. R. Bond, J. E. Charlton, and C. J. Woolf), p. 255. Elsevier Science, Amsterdam; with permission).

It is known that peptides associated with C-fibres are present in low concentrations at birth but increase rapidly in the first 2 weeks of life (Fitzgerald and Gibson 1984). Receptor populations in the substantia gelatinosa are also different at birth and do not follow the adult pattern for several weeks postnatally. Maturation of opioid pathways as evidenced by receptor population does not begin until after the first postnatal week (Barr *et al.* 1986). There is evidence to suggest that slowly reacting pain pathways involving neuropeptides are present at birth and that faster pathways in C-fibres do not develop until about a week postnatally.

This raises a fundamental and interesting concept. The neonatal period is traditionally defined as the first 4 weeks of life, but should we now seek to modify this in the light of these findings, at least as far as pain pathways are concerned? From experimental evidence, and clinical observation, the 1 week full-term neonate is a different animal from the 4 week neonate. A full-term baby of 4 weeks, although not having mature hepatic enzyme systems, does appear to possess a different 'opioid receptor configuration' from the 1- or 2-day-old. Ex-premature neonates do seem to be more at risk from exogenous opioid administration.

From the work of Fitzgerald and others it seems likely that painful stimuli may not provoke the usual response seen in adults and older children, but rather alter the behaviour of the neonate producing somewhat unpredictable responses. Because the neospinothalamic tracts develop later, pain may be more difficult to localize and the responses less specific.


## FETAL PAIN

Intrauterine operations on the fetus are frequently undertaken without provision of analgesia as many doctors have taken the view that the fetus is too immature to feel pain. This, of course, is analogous to previous thinking concerning the neonate.

A recent study (Giannakoulopoulos *et al.* 1994) of 187 procedures has demonstrated that the fetus mounts a stress response to intra-abdominal fetal blood sampling, as evidenced by increases in fetal plasma cortisol and $\beta$-endorphin. The available data suggest that the 'stress response' as evidenced by the rise in adrenocortical hormones in adults and in amniotic fluid correlates closely with rises in $\beta$-endorphin. However, these observations still do not prove that fetuses feel pain, but lend weight to the assumption that if neuro-hormonal pathways are developed early in gestation, there exists at least the possibility that the fetus may experience pain, and that the vigorous breathing and limb movement observed during fetal operations are indeed a response to pain.

Such arguments may compel us to believe that adequate analgesia must therefore be provided for even the most premature and sick neonate. It appears that the stress response itself is not directly linked to pain, in that when pain is controlled by epidural analgesia, the stress response is still observed and cannot therefore be used as a quantitative measure of analgesia. Further, it has not yet been shown conclusively that ablation of the stress response has a beneficial effect on outcome. It has been shown, however, that epidural analgesia is more effective than systemic opioids in blunting the hormonal response to stress in infants (Wolf et al. 1992).

## THERAPEUTIC APPROACHES

From our increased understanding of the behaviour of small infants toward pain there has been a growing awareness amongst those looking after children that we can no longer leave pain untreated in this group just because they do not behave as though they are feeling pain in the same way as an older child or adult. The small infant's response to pain is complex and unpredictable, it is therefore particularly difficult to measure. Because of this, we think it prudent to assume that all surgical procedures produce residual pain which should be treated appropriately. This may simply be with paracetamol or other mild analgesics, but frequently the magnitude of the surgery will require opioid analgesia or nerve blockade with a local anaesthetic agent.

### Local anaesthetic agents

Local anaesthetic (or analgesic) agents are primarily used to block nerve impulses in pain pathways, but because they affect all excitable tissue they also cause motor and autonomic block, the effect of which may be useful during operative procedures. However, myocardial depression and convulsions can occur with inadvertent intravascular injection. Bupivacaine is particularly cardiotoxic, whereas the central nervous system toxicity of lignocaine and prilocaine exceeds the cardiotoxicity.

*Pharmacokinetics*

Of more concern to us when discussing the use of these agents in children are the pharmacokinetics of local anaesthetics, particularly with regard to toxicity and the fate of the drug in the very young.

Following absorption, these drugs are widely distributed throughout the body and may have systemic effects if the unbound fraction is high enough. There are marked differences, especially in babies, in the pharmacokinetics and pharmacodynamics of these agents compared with the adult.

Because local anaesthetics are highly protein-bound, the *plasma* concentration generally exceeds that of whole blood (Tucker and Mather 1975, 1979). As the plasma concentration of the drug increases, there is a marked *decrease* in the fraction bound. For example, for bupivacaine, at 2 $\mu$g ml$^{-1}$ *free base* in plasma, 95 per cent is protein bound. This decreases at 20 $\mu$g ml$^{-1}$ to 65 per cent. Since the unbound fraction is that available to exert the clinical effects of the drug, and also for metabolism and excretion, it can be seen that protein binding has great relevance to the toxicity of the drug (Tucker *et al.* 1970). If greater doses of local anaesthetic are used, the free fraction is increased with increased potential for toxic effects. The minimum dose which will exert the required effect should therefore be used.

There are two main groups of local anaesthetic agents, the esters and the amides. The ester group comprises:

(1)  benzocaine;
(2)  chloroprocaine;
(3)  cocaine;
(4)  procaine; and
(5)  amethocaine.

Cocaine is still widely used for topical anaesthesia in older children and adults, since, unlike other local anaesthetics in common use, it produces marked local vasoconstriction, which is particularly useful in ENT surgery.

Amide anaesthetics are:

(1)  lignocaine;
(2)  prilocaine;
(3)  bupivacaine;

(4)  etidocaine;
(5)  mepivacaine; and
(6)  ropivacaine.

Lignocaine, prilocaine, and bupivacaine are the most favoured agents in the UK. Ropivacaine has been shown to have a more rapid distribution phase with plasma levels falling more rapidly than those of racemic bupivacaine (Arthur *et al.* 1988).

Bupivacaine, ropivacaine, and mepivacaine appear to be equipotent in directly inhibiting cyclic AMP (cAMP) in muscle, but this direct inhibition may not actually be of great importance in clinical cardiac toxicity (Butterworth *et al.* 1993). It has been demonstrated that the concentration of local anaesthetic agent which reduces adrenaline-induced cAMP production fits quite closely with the relative toxicity levels generally quoted in the literature (Butterworth and Pang 1992). Ropivacaine is clinically similar to bupivacaine but is less arrhythmogenic and produces a less depressant effect on cardiac muscle after comparable convulsive doses in dogs (Feldman *et al.* 1991).

The rate of uptake of local anaesthetic into the nerve cell depends on the lipid solubility of the unionized molecule. Only the unionized molecule will pass through the cell membrane into the neurone. As the ionized form becomes unionized, some of the fraction bound to protein becomes unbound. Local anaesthetic agents usually possess $pK_a$ values which are higher than the pH of plasma or neuronal tissues, and at equilibrium most of the drug is in the ionized state. The ionized form is more water-soluble, thus aiding diffusion, but poor lipid solubility prevents the ionized form from crossing cell membranes easily. The more lipid-soluble compounds (e.g. bupivacaine) have greater anaesthetic potency.

A large proportion of the drug will also be bound to protein so that only a small, free, unionized fraction of the dose actually penetrates into the cell. Diffusion into the nerve cell membrane seems to be greater in small children, thus lower concentrations of local anaesthetic agent are needed to produce a block compared to adults (Warner *et al.* 1987).

The effect of local anaesthetics depends not only on penetration across the nerve membrane but also on the number of nodes of Ranvier that are blocked. Impulses can 'jump' or partially depolarize several nodes. The distances over which the local anaesthetic is effective will also determine the nature of the block. If myelination is incomplete, the nodes are closer and the membrane is blocked with less volume and concentration.

Local anaesthetics are mostly bound to albumin in the plasma and alpha$_1$ acid glycoprotein in the extracellular fluid generally (Denson *et al.* 1984). They also bind to erythrocytes, which may be more important in neonates than in older children.

Amide-type local anaesthetics bind strongly to alpha$_1$ acid glycoprotein but have less affinity for albumin. The greater quantities of albumin present, however, make it an important binding protein, but disturbances of albumin concentration only become significant when the concentration of local anaesthetic agent is high (e.g. for bupivacaine, 10 $\mu$g ml$^{-1}$, a figure not normally encountered in clinical practice).

However, increases in the amount of alpha$_1$ acid glycoprotein, such as is found in some oncology patients, will greatly reduce the free fraction of bupivacaine. Clearance is also reduced but systemic toxicity does not readily occur because of the increased binding capacity. Neonates have lower concentrations of both albumin and alpha$_1$ acid glycoprotein, being about 60 per cent of the adult concentration for albumin and 30 per cent for alpha$_1$ acid glycoprotein. This reduction in binding capacity for local anaesthetics will increase the free (unbound) fraction *for any given dose* and thus increase the possibility of toxic effects.

In a study (Mazoit *et al.* 1988) involving caudal injection of bupivacaine in 13 infants aged 1–6 months of age, Mazoit *et al.* found peak serum concentrations of between 0.55 and 1.93 $\mu$g ml$^{-1}$, the time taken to reach the peak ranging from 10 to 60 minutes. Terminal half-life (mean) was 7.7 hours ($\pm$ SD 2.4 h). The free fraction (measured in 11 infants) was increased when compared to the adult value, and the negative correlation with age was highly significant.

Alpha$_1$ acid glycoprotein levels correlated significantly with age in this study, whereas albumin levels did not. Terminal half-life and distribution volume at steady state exceeded the values reported by Ecoffey *et al.* for children aged between 5.5 and 10 years (Ecoffey *et al.* 1985a; Mazoit *et al.* 1988). Mazoit *et al.* postulate that the increased volume of distribution of hydrophilic drugs (bupivacaine 80 per cent ionized at pH 7.40) decreases from birth to adulthood. Because of the large extracellular fluid volume in neonates and small infants (total body water 80 per cent of body weight), local anaesthetic agents have a larger distribution volume than in the older child or adult (Marselli *et al.* 1980; Ecoffey *et al.* 1985a). The mean time to reach peak serum concentration in the study of Mazoit *et al.* was similar to that in older children.

Binding to fat plays an important role in the pharmacokinetics of local anaesthetic drugs. Small children have less epidural fat and so local anaesthetic agents are absorbed form the epidural space earlier than in adults, the duration of block is shorter and the peak plasma concentration higher.

### Clearance

All local anaesthetic agents, both esters and amides, undergo metabolic change so that only a very small fraction is excreted unchanged. In neonates, the rate of metabolism is slower than that in adults for several agents but lignocaine seems to be little affected. Low cardiac output states reduce hepatic clearance due to the effect on hepatic and portal venous blood flow.

Ester-type local anaesthetics are metabolized by plasma cholinesterases. Intravascular injections cause disproportionate toxic effects because of the high peak concentration at the heart and brain. Furthermore, the rate of delivery exceeds the metabolic capacity of the plasma enzymes.

Neonates do not have the same capacity for ester hydrolysis as older children because plasma cholinesterase activity increases during the first few months of life and is decreased in the premature. This has given rise to some concern over the use of amethocaine cream in small babies. Significant concentrations may cross the placenta.

Amethocaine cream applied to intact skin prior to venepuncture produces very little measurable amethocaine in plasma. However, as with EMLA® cream, care must be taken not only to apply such cream to abraded skin or mucosal surfaces where absorption may be very rapid.

Amides undergo phase I (oxidation) and phase II (conjugation) metabolism by liver microsomal enzymes. Some of the metabolites also possess local anaesthetic actions. Slow renal excretion of these polar metabolites is thought to be responsible for toxicity in some patients with poor renal function. The neonate appears to possess the necessary enzyme systems for these reactions to take place but the capacity of the system to handle the drug load is much less than in older children. Despite the higher cardiac output, infants demonstrate a reduced clearance of all amide local anaesthetics, due principally to reduced capacity for phase I pathways. This is a very important consideration when using bupivacaine in neonates, and bupivacaine is probably the most commonly used agent for regional anaesthesia in the UK.

Bupivacaine (unlike, for example, lignocaine) is almost as cardiotoxic as neurotoxic and may produce profound myocardial depression without much neuroexcitatory effect, that is, before twitching can be observed clinically. Absorption, and therefore maximal plasma concentration and toxicity, can be reduced if low concentrations of adrenaline are used in the solution (e.g. 1 in 200 000).

The lipophilic free base is easily able to cross the blood–brain barrier. Those agents which have greater potency are generally more lipophilic (etidocaine being a possible exception) and are also more toxic to the central nervous system (CNS). CNS toxicity is dose dependent, with initial sedation giving rise to excitability and convulsions, finally followed by coma and respiratory arrest.

## Use of opioids with local anaesthetics

Opioids, particularly morphine, diamorphine, and fentanyl, are now widely used in epidural anaesthesia in children. Intrathecal morphine is also sometimes used (Jones *et al*. 1984).

Opioid receptors are present in high numbers in the spinal cord, and administration of opioids, either epidurally or intrathecally, can achieve potent analgesia with small doses. This analgesia is both more profound and longer lasting than comparable doses given systemically. Both visceral and somatic afferents are blocked (Covino 1986).

Side-effects include respiratory depression, nausea and vomiting, itching, and urinary retention. These features are more common after intrathecal as opposed to epidural administration, probably due to rostral spread of the opioid in the cerebrospinal fluid. Respiratory depression and pruritus can be abolished by titrated infusion of naloxone, while still allowing adequate analgesia.

The development of analgesia following epidural administration of 50 $\mu$g kg$^{-1}$ of morphine takes 30 minutes (Ecoffey *et al.* 1985b) and lasts up to 24 hours. Intrathecal administration results in a faster onset time (5–15 minutes). Administration of 20 $\mu$g kg$^{-1}$ of intrathecal morphine will produce analgesia lasting many hours. Respiratory depression may be significant and is said to be maximal at about 4 hours after an intrathecal dose. Some authors recommend that intrathecal morphine should not be given within 4 hours of systemically administered opioids (Samii *et al.* 1981).

## Clonidine

Clonidine is an $\alpha_2$ adrenoceptor agonist. It acts in the dorsal horn of the spinal cord to stimulate $\alpha_2$ adrenergic receptors. It causes analgesia by inhibiting release of substance P. Both pre- and post-synaptic $\alpha_2$ adrenergic receptors exist. Stimulation of these receptors decreases release of noradrenaline from nerve terminals. The analgesia produced by clonidine is reduced by atropine and enhanced by neostigmine (Gordh *et al.* 1989).

Clonidine given intrathecally may produce bradycardia. The effect can be minimized by intrathecal pretreatment with neo-stigmine which increases spinal sympathetic preganglionic activity, which in turn tends to increase blood pressure. Experimental work suggests that this combination approach would produce minimal side-effects (Williams *et al.* 1992). Due to the direct effect on sympathetic outflow, there is a more marked fall in the blood pressure after thoracic, compared with lumbar epidural, clonidine (Eisenach and Tong 1991).

Clonidine produces sedation whether it is administered sys-temically or spinally. A study of children aged 1–10 years undergoing orthopaedic surgery demonstrated prolonged analge-sia from a clonidine/bupivacaine mixture given for caudal epidural block compared to bupivacaine alone (mean duration 9.8 v. 5.2 hours). The clonidine group, given 2 $\mu$g kg$^{-1}$ with 0.25 per cent bupivacaine 1 ml kg$^{-1}$, showed significantly longer postoperative sedation (Lee and Rubin 1994).

Clonidine does not produce nausea, respiratory depression, urinary retention or itching, which is associated with intrathecal

epidural or systemic opioids, and therefore has potential for sup-
plementation of central neural blocks. Extradural clonidine does
reduce the ventilatory response to carbon dioxide (Penlon *et al.*
1991) and, with the central sedation that occurs, has the potential
to cause respiratory depression, which must be considered seri-
ously in very young children, particularly those with immature
control systems. The combination of local anaesthetic agents and
clonidine seems suitable for quite small children (1 year of age)
but more work needs to be done before it can be recommended
for routine use in babies.

## REFERENCES

Altman, J. and Bayer, S. A. (1984). The development of the rat spinal
cord. *Advances in Anatomy Embryology and Cell Biology*, **85**, 166.

Anand, K. J. S. and Hickey, P. R. (1987). Pain and its effects in the
human neonate and fetus. *New England Journal of Medicine*, **317**,
1321–9.

Arthur, G. R., Feldman, H. S., and Covino, B. C. (1988). Comparative
pharmacokinetics of bupivacaine and ropivacaine, a new amide local
anesthetic. *Anesthesia Analgesia*, **67**, 1053–8.

Barr, G. A., Paredes, W., Erickson, K. L., and Zukin, R. S. (1986).
Kappa-opioid receptor mediated analgesia in the developing rat.
*Developmental Brain Research*, **29**, 145–52.

Bicknell, H. R. and Beal, J. A. (1984). Axonal and dendritic neurons in
the lumbosacral spinal cord of the rat. *Journal of Comparative
Neurology*, **226**, 508–22.

Butterworth, J. F., and Pang, J. H. (1992). Inhibition of $\beta$-adrenergic
receptor binding by mepivacaine, ropivacaine and bupivacaine.
Anesthesiology, **77**, A846.

Butterworth, J. F. *et al.* (1993). Bupivacaine inhibits cyclic $3'5'$ adeno-
sine monophosphate production. *Anesthesiology*, **79**, 88–95.

Chan, C. W. Y., and Dallaire, M. (1989). Subjective pain sensation is
linearly correlated with the flexion reflex in man. *Brain Research*, **479**,
145–50.

Charnay, Y., Paulin, C., Dray, F., and Dubois, P. N. (1984).
Distribution of enkephalin in human foetus and infant spinal cord: an
immunofluorescence study. *Journal of Comparative Neurology*, **223**,
415–23.

Charnay, Y. *et al.* (1987). Ontogeny of somatostatin-like immuno-
reactivity in the human foetus and spinal cord. *Developmental Brain
Research*, **36**, 63–73.

Covino, B. G. (1986). Epidural morphine provides postoperative pain relief in peripheral vascular and orthopaedic surgical patients: A dose-response study. *Anesthesia Analgesia*, **65**, 165–70.

Denson, D. D., Coyle, D. E., Thompson, G. A., and Myers, J. A. (1984). The role of alpha₁ acid glycoprotein and albumin in human serum binding of bupivacaine. *Clinical Pharmacology and Therapeutics*, **35**, 409–16.

Devries, J. I. P., Visser, G. H. A., and Prechtl, H. F. R. (1982). The emergence of fetal behaviour. I. Qualitative aspects. *Early Human Development*, 7, 301–22.

Ecoffey, C. *et al.* (1985*a*). Bupivacaine in children. Pharmacokinetics following caudal anesthesia. *Anesthesiology*, **63**, 447–8.

Ecoffey, C., Attia, J., and Samii, K. (1985*b*). Analgesia and side-effects following epidural morphine in children. *Anesthesiology*, **63**, A470.

Eisenach J. C. and Tong, C. (1991). Site of hemodynamic effects of intrathecal adrenergic agonists. *Anesthesiology*, **74**, 766–71.

Ekholm, J. (1987). Postnatal changes in cutaneous reflexes and in the discharge pattern of cutaneous and particular sense organs. *Acta Physiologica Scandinavica (Suppl.)*, **297**, 1–130.

Feldman, H. S. *et al.* (1991). Treatment of acute systemic toxicity after the rapid intravenous injection of ropivacaine and bupivacaine in the conscious dog. *Anesthesia Analgesia*, **73**, 373–84.

Fitzgerald, M. (1991). In *Proceedings of the VI World Congress on Pain*, pp. 253–61. Elsevier Science, Amsterdam.

Fitzgerald, M. and Gibson, S. (1984). The postnatal physiological and neurochemical development of peripheral sensory C-fibres. *Neuroscience*, **13**, 933–44.

Fitzgerald, M., Shaw, A., and Mackintosh, N. (1987). The postnatal development of the flexor reflex: a comparative study in premature infants and newborn rat pups. *Developmental Medicine and Child Neurology*, **30**, 520–6.

Fitzgerald, M., Millard, C., and MacIntosh, N. (1988). Hyperalgesia in premature infants. *Lancet*, **i**, 292.

Fitzgerald, M., Reynolds, M. L., and Benowitz, L. I. (1991). GAP-43 expression in the developing rat lumbar spinal cord. *Neuroscience*, **41**, 187–99.

Forger, N. G. and Breedlove, S. M. (1987). Motoneuronal death during human fetal development. *Journal of Comparative Neurology*, **264**, 11–122.

Giannakoulopoulos, X., Sepulveda, W., Kourtis, P., and Fisk, N. M. (1994). Fetal plasma cortisol and β-endorphin response to intrauterine needling. *Lancet*, **344**, 77–81.

Gordh, T. *et al.* (1989). Interactions between noradrenergic and cholinergic mechanisms involved in spinal noiceptive processing. *Acta Anaesthesiologica Scandinavica*, **33**, 39–47.

Hooker, D. (1952). *The prenatal origin of behaviour.* University of Kansas Press, Lawrence, Kansas.

Jones, S. E. F. *et al.* (1984). Intrathecal morphine for post-operative pain relief in children. *British Journal of Anaesthesia,* **56**, 137–40.

Klimach, V. J. and Cooke, R. W. I. (1988). Maturation of the neonatal somatosensory evoked response in preterm infants. *Developmental Medicine and Child Neurology,* **30**, 208–14.

Lee, J. J. and Rubin, A. P. (1994). Comparison of a bupivacaine-clonidine mixture with plain bupivacaine for caudal analgesia in children. *British Journal of Anaesthesia,* **72**, 258–62.

McGrath, P. J. and Unruh, A. M. (1987). Pain in children and adolescents. *Pain Research and Clinical Management,* V1.

Marselli, P. L., Franco-Marselli, R., and Bossi, L. (1980). Clinical pharmacokinetics in newborns and infants: age-related differences and therapeutic implications. *Clinical Pharmacokinetics,* **5**, 485–527.

Marti, E., Gibson, S. J., and Polak, J. M. (1987). Ontogeny of peptide and amino-containing neurons in motor, sensory and autonomic regions of rat and human spinal cord. *Journal of Comparative Neurology,* **266**, 332–59.

Mazoit, J. X., Denson, D. D., and Samii, K. (1988). Pharmacokinetics of bupivacaine following caudal anaesthesia in infants. *Anesthesiology,* **68**, 387–91.

Mrzljak, L., Uylings, H. B. M., Kostovic, I., and Van Eden, C. G. (1988). Prenatal development of neurons in the human prefrontal cortex: a qualitative golgi study. *Journal of Comparative Neurology,* **271**, 355–86.

Narayanan, C. H., Fox, M. W., and Hamburger, C. (1971). Prenatal development of spontaneous and evoked activity in the rat. *Behaviour,* **40**, 100–34.

Okado, N. and Kojima, T. (1984). Ontogeny of the central nervous system: neurogenesis, fibre connection, synaptogenesis and myelination in the spinal cord. In *Continuity of neural functions from prenatal to post-natal life,* (ed. H. F. R. Prechtl). *Clinical and Developmental Medicine,* **94**, 79–92.

Oppenheim, R. W. (1987). The absence of significant post-natal mo-torneuron death in the brachial and lumbar spinal cord of the rat. *Journal of Comparative Neurology,* **246**, 281–6.

Penon, C., Ecoffey, C., and Cohen, S. E. (1991). Ventilatory response to carbon dioxide after epidural clonidine injection. *Anesthesia and Analgesia,* **72**, 761–4.

Samii, K., Chaurin, A. A., and Viars, P. (1981). Postoperative spinal analgesia with morphine. *British Journal of Anaesthesia,* **53**, 817–20.

Thairu, B. K. (1971). Postnatal changes in the somaesthetic evoked potentials of the albino rat. *Nature,* **231**, 30–1.

Tucker, G. T. and Mather, L. E. (1975). Pharmacokinetics of local anaesthetic agents. *British Journal of Anaesthesia,* **47**, 213–24.

Tucker, G. T. and Mather, L. E. (1979). Clinical pharmacokinetics of local anaesthetics. *Clinical Pharmacokinetics*, **4**, 241–78.

Tucker, G. T., Boyes, R. N., Bridenbaugh, P. O., and Moore, D. C. (1970). Binding of anilide-type local anesthetics in human plasma: I. Relationship between binding, physiochemical properties and anesthetic activity. *Anesthesiology*, **33**, 287–303.

Vaughan, J. E. and Grieshaber, S. A. (1973). A morphological investigation of an early reflex pathway in developing rat spinal cord. *Journal of Comparative Neurology*, **148**, 177–210.

Warner, M. A. *et al.* (1987). The effects of age, epinephrine and operative site on duration of caudal analgesia in pediatric patients. *Anesthesia Analgesia*, **66**, 995–8.

Williams, J. S., Tong, C., and Eisenach, J. C. (1992). Neostigmine counteracts spinal clonidine–induced hypotension in sheep. *Anesthesiology*, **78**, 301–7.

Wise, S. P. and Jones, E. G. (1978). Developmental studies of thalamo-cortical and commissural connections in the rat somatic sensory cortex. *Journal of Comparative Neurology*, **178**, 187–208.

Wolf, A. R. *et al.* (1992). Effect of extradural analgesia on stress responses to abdominal surgery in infants. *British Journal of Anaesthesia*, **70**, 654–60.

# Part 2

# Techniques of regional anaesthesia: topical and infiltration anaesthesia

# 3

# *Topical anaesthesia of skin and mucous membranes*

## J. M. PEUTRELL

## ANATOMY

### Skin

Skin consists of two zones:

(1) the epidermis;
(2) the dermis.

The epidermis is a stratified epithelium without nerve endings or blood vessels. It consists of several distinct layers. The outer horny layer of skin is called the stratum corneum and over most of the body surface is 75–100 $\mu$m thick. It is a dense layer consisting of cells containing mainly keratin and extracellular tissue with a high lipid content. The dermis is a vascular layer with specialized pain receptors (nociceptors) lying at, or, just above the dermo-epidermal junction.

Cutaneous pain receptors are probably formed from free nerve endings. They are of two principal types:

(1) mechanical nociceptors responding to pinprick, squeezing, and crushing;
(2) thermal nociceptors responding to severe mechanical stimuli and hot and cold temperatures.

### Mucous membranes

The mucous membranes of the oro-pharynx and trachea are thin and have no cornified layer. Histological characteristics differ between sites: the mouth is lined with stratified squamous, the nose with columnar or pseudostratified, and the trachea with pseudostratified ciliated epithelium. Sensory receptors lie beneath or within the membranes. Uptake of local anaesthetics across mucous membranes is very rapid.

## IDEAL CHARACTERISTICS OF PREPARATIONS FOR TOPICAL ANAESTHESIA OF THE SKIN

The clinical characteristics of local anaesthetics applied to the skin are influenced by their bioavailability and rate of delivery to the nerve cell membrane. The stratum corneum is the main barrier to the absorption of drugs. It has a high lipid content and is more easily penetrated by lipophilic drugs.

Local anaesthetics are weak bases usually rendered water-soluble by producing salts (e.g. hydrochloride or sulphate). Water-soluble preparations are poorly absorbed across cornified epithelium but are absorbed rapidly across mucous membranes and open wounds. Pure preparations of free bases of local anaesthetics exist as oils or amorphous solids with low melting points. They are poorly soluble in water but very soluble in lipids and, if liquid, diffuse more easily across the lipid-rich stratum corneum than ionized forms.

The ideal characteristics of formulations used for topical anaesthesia of the skin are:

(1)  the local anaesthetic should exist as a liquid or solution at body temperature;

(2)  the formulation should contain a high concentration of lipophilic base that will penetrate the epidermis rapidly;

(3)  the local anaesthetic base should have a high lipid solubility;

(4)  the base should have a higher affinity for the skin than the formulation;

(5)  the formulation should have the lowest effective concentration of free base but in an adequate concentration to promote penetration of the skin and decrease the latency of onset;

(6)  the base should not have a such a high affinity for the stratum corneum that it will not diffuse into the dermis; and

(7)  the formulation should not produce hypersensitivity reactions or systemic toxicity.

The stratum corneum can act as a reservoir for topical anaesthetics, and analgesia often continues to develop after the local anaesthetic preparation has been removed. Covering the site of application with a occlusive dressing promotes penetration of the skin.

## FURTHER READING

Woolfson, D. and McCafferty, D. (1993). *Percutaneous local anaesthesia.* Ellis Horwood, New York.

## DRUGS USED FOR TOPICAL ANAESTHESIA

Only three preparations of local anaesthetics are suitable for topical anaesthesia of intact skin: lignocaine base in high concentration (e.g. 30 per cent), eutectic mixture of local anaesthetics (EMLA®, Astra), and amethocaine (e.g. Ametop®, Smith & Nephew). Preparations of free base (e.g. lignocaine, amethocaine, and EMLA) and solutions of salts of local anaesthetics (e.g. lignocaine, cocaine, and amethocaine) are effective anaesthetics for wounds or mucous membranes.

### Amethocaine (tetracaine)

Amethocaine is an ester local anaesthetic used for anaesthesia of skin, wounds, and corneal epithelium. It is metabolized by plasma cholinesterases. Atypical enzymes probably hydrolyse amethocaine as rapidly as normal cholinesterases.

### *Anaesthesia of the skin*

Amethocaine base is more lipophilic than either lignocaine or prilocaine bases. It is more potent, has a longer duration of anaesthesia, and, in appropriate formulation, penetrates the stratum corneum more rapidly than EMLA.

Only diffusible amethocaine base is absorbed across the stratum corneum. Aqueous solutions contain a reduced amount of free base because a proportion will become ionized. Amethocaine can be dissolved in inert oil (as a solution or an oil-in-water emulsion) but the relatively high affinity for the formulation will reduce uptake into the skin. Solutions of amethocaine in water or oil must be prepared in unacceptably high concentrations to obtain significant analgesia of the skin.

Smith & Nephew have developed a 4 per cent preparation of amethocaine for anaesthesia of the skin before venepuncture or cannulation. It is available as Ametop®. In the presence of moisture, the melting point of the free base of amethocaine is reduced from around 40 °C to 30 °C, producing an oily liquid. Amethocaine base can be formulated as an aqueous suspension of solid amethocaine (a gel). At body temperature the amethocaine melts to produce oil droplets. The amethocaine is then in a diffusible form with a relatively low affinity for the formulation and anaesthesia of the skin can be obtained with acceptable concentrations. Ametop produces analgesia of the skin within 30–45 minutes that lasts about 4 hours. A self-adhesive patch of anhydrous amethocaine producing an equally rapid onset of anaesthesia has also been developed but is not available for clinical use. The amethocaine becomes hydrated at the skin–patch interface and melts to form an oil droplet suspension from which local anaesthetic can diffuse into the skin.

Amethocaine is slowly absorbed into the systemic circulation across intact skin and is rapidly metabolized by tissue and plasma cholinesterases before plasma concentrations can rise. It may produce vasodilatation in some children; this may be helpful for venous cannulation. Some patients complain of itching at the site of application that resolves when amethocaine is removed.

### Mucous membranes and cornea

Amethocaine is very rapidly absorbed across mucous membranes and is no longer used to provide anaesthesia of the tracheo-bronchial tree in the UK because of the risks of toxicity (including asystole and ventricular fibrillation).

Amethocaine hydrochloride solutions (0.5 and 1.0 per cent) are commonly used to provide topical anaesthesia of the corneal epithelium.

## Wounds

Amethocaine 0.5 per cent can be combined with adrenaline and cocaine as TAC (tetracaine (amethocaine)) 0.5 per cent, adrenaline 1 : 2000, cocaine 11.8 per cent) and applied to minor skin wounds to provide anaesthesia before suturing (see below).

## FURTHER READING

Freeman, J. A., Doyle, E., Tee Im, N. G., and Morton, N. S. (1993). Topical anaesthesia of the skin: a review. *Paediatric Anaesthesia*, **3**, 129–38.
Woolfson, D., and McCafferty, D. (1993). *Percutaneous local anaesthesia.* Ellis Horwood, New York.

## REFERENCES

Doyle, E., Freeman, J., Im, N.T., and Morton, N.S. (1993). An evaluation of a new self-adhesive patch preparation of amethocaine for topical anaesthesia prior to venous cannulation in children. *Anaesthesia*, **48**, 1050–2.
McCafferty, D. F., and Woolfson, A. D. (1993). New patch delivery system for percutaneous local anaesthesia. *British Journal of Anaesthesia*, **71**, 370–4.
McCafferty, D. F., Woolfson, A. D., and Boston, V. (1989). *In vivo* assessment of percutaneous local anaesthetic preparations. *British Journal of Anaesthesia*, **62**, 17–21.
Mazumdar, B., Tomlinson, A. A., and Faulder, G. C. (1991). Preliminary study to assay plasma amethocaine concentrations after topical application of a new local anaesthetic cream containing amethocaine. *British Journal of Anaesthesia*, **67**, 432–6.
Woolfson, A. D., McCafferty, D. F., McClelland, K.H., and Boston, V. (1988). Concentration–response analysis of percutaneous local anaesthetic formulations. *British Journal of Anaesthesia*, **61**, 589–92.
Woolfson, A. D., McCafferty, D. F., and Boston, V. (1990). Clinical experiences with a novel percutaneous amethocaine preparation: prevention of pain due to venepuncture in children. *British Journal of Clinical Pharmacology*, **30**, 273–9.

## Cocaine

Cocaine is an ester of benzoic acid that has local anaesthetic and sympathomimetic properties. It is used to provide topical anaesthesia and vasoconstriction of mucous membranes, particularly of the nose. Cocaine can be mixed with adrenaline and amethocaine (tetracaine) to produce TAC (tetracaine 0.5 per cent, adrenaline 1 : 2000, cocaine 11.8 per cent) which can be applied to minor wounds to provide anaesthesia for suturing (see below).

Cocaine is never given systemically because of toxicity.

### Dose

The maximum dose recommended for topical application in adults is 1.5 mg kg$^{-1}$. Toxicity has been reported in a baby given 0.7 mg kg$^{-1}$ intranasally and cocaine should be used very cautiously in small children. Cocaine is usually prepared as 4 or 10 per cent solutions (40–100 mg ml$^{-1}$) and the volumes that can be used safely are very small and must be measured carefully.

### Complications

#### Central nervous system toxicity

Cocaine initially stimulates the central nervous system producing euphoria, hallucinations, hyper-reflexia, convulsions, dilated pupils, hyperventilation, and hyperpyrexia. In later stages cocaine depresses the central nervous system, producing coma and ventilatory depression.

#### Cardiovascular toxicity

Cocaine blocks the re-uptake of catecholamines at adrenergic nerve endings, potentiating the effects of circulating catecholamines and sympathetic stimulation. The cardiovascular features of cocaine toxicity include: vasoconstriction, tachycardia, arrhythmias, and hypertension.

Toxic signs and symptoms may persist for several hours because of continuing absorption across vasoconstricted membranes.

Treatment includes:

(1) removing any remaining cocaine by rinsing with water,
(2) anticonvulsants (e.g. Diazemuls® 0.25 mg kg$^{-1}$ intravenously),
(3) $\alpha$- and $\beta$-blockers (e.g. labetalol 0.2 mg kg$^{-1}$ intravenously repeated every 5 minutes according to response).

## REFERENCES

Schou, H., Krogh, B., and Knudsen, F. (1987). Unexpected cocaine intoxication in a fourteen month old child following topical administration. *Clinical Toxicology*, **25**, 419–22.

Schubert, C. J., and Wason, S. (1992). Cocaine toxicity in an infant following intranasal instillation of a four per cent cocaine solution. *Pediatric Emergency Care*, **8**, 82–3.

### Eutectic mixture of local anaesthetics (EMLA®)

Lignocaine and prilocaine bases have melting points of 67 °C and 37 °C, respectively, and are waxy solids at room temperature. When mixed together there is no chemical interaction between the molecules but the melting points of the bases are reduced. The word 'eutectic' describes this phenomenon. A mixture of equal amounts of lignocaine and prilocaine has a melting point of about 18 °C and forms a runny oil at room temperature.

EMLA® (eutectic mixture of local anaesthetics, Astra Pharmaceuticals Ltd) is an oil-in-water emulsion containing lignocaine 25 mg g$^{-1}$ and prilocaine 25 mg g$^{-1}$ (Fig. 3.1). The pH of the formulation is 9.4, ensuring that virtually all the local anaesthetic molecules are unionized. The concentration of each local anaesthetic within the emulsion is 2.5 per cent, but the oil droplets consist of 80 per cent unionized local anaesthetic.

When applied to skin, the lipophilic bases of the local anaesthetics permeate the stratum corneum to form a depot from which they diffuse into the dermis to produce anaesthesia. EMLA abolishes pain sensation before warmth, touch, and non-painful pinprick. The onset and duration of analgesia depend upon skin thickness and vascularity: a high blood flow or thin skin (e.g. premature babies) increase the onset and reduce the duration of anaesthesia. The rate uptake of local anaesthetic across diseased skin (e.g. eczema) is greater but the duration of analgesia is shorter.

EMLA is supplied in tubes containing 5 or 30 g. One to two grams are applied to approximately 10 cm² of skin, which is then covered with a transparent occlusive dressing (e.g. Tegaderm®). The maximum areas of application for different weights of children are shown in Table 3.1.

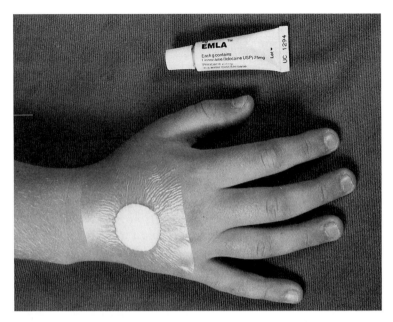

**Fig. 3.1** EMLA® cream (Astra): in a 5 g tube (above), and applied to the back of the hand (below).

**Table 3.1** Maximum application areas of EMLA cream in children (Gajraj *et al.* 1994)

| Body weight (kg) | Maximum area of skin (cm²) |
|---|---|
| < 10 | 100 |
| 10–20 | 600 |
| > 20 | 2000 |

EMLA must be applied for a minimum of 60 minutes to provide reliable anaesthesia for venepuncture in children aged 4–17 years. The minimum time of application is shorter (i.e. 30 minutes) in younger children. If EMLA is applied for less than 120 minutes, the density of anaesthesia increases for 30–60 minutes after removal because uptake of local anaesthetic into the dermis continues from the stratum corneum. EMLA applied for less than 2.5 hours can produce skin blanching but longer application tends to produce erythema. This is explained by the slow rate of accumulation of local anaesthetics within the vascular layers of skin, producing concentrations that are initially low but which then rise. Low concentrations of lignocaine and prilocaine are vasoconstrictors but high concentrations are vasodilators.

A single application of 5 g of EMLA in children aged 1–6 years produces a small rise in the plasma concentration of methaemoglobin, although the total concentration remains within normal limits. In normal babies aged 3–12 months EMLA 2 g produces very low plasma concentrations of lignocaine and prilocaine, and a clinically insignificant increase in methaemoglobin concentration. Children with pre-existing disease (e.g. anaemia, congenital or idiopathic methaemoglobinaemia, those taking sulphonamide antibiotics) or very permeable skin (e.g. small or premature babies) may be at risk of developing methaemoglobinaemia induced by prilocaine, particularly after frequent applications.

## Indications

### Anaesthesia of the skin
EMLA can be used to provide anaesthesia for some minor operations and procedures in children including:

(1)  intravenous cannulation;
(2)  phlebotomy;
(3)  injection into implanted ports of central venous cannulae;
(4)  lumbar puncture;
(5)  cautery, curettage, and debridement of skin lesions (e.g. laser treatment for port-wine stain, removal of molluscum contagiosum);
(6)  renal biopsy;
(7)  separation of preputial adhesions; and
(8)  skin grafting.

EMLA has also been used in adults to provide anaesthesia for:

(1)  cannulation of kidney dialysis fistulae;
(2)  arterial cannulation;
(3)  insertion of grommets into the tympanic membrane.

### Anaesthesia of gingival mucosa
EMLA produces anaesthesia of the gingival mucosa within about 5 minutes and can be used to reduce the pain of regional block for

dental surgery. It has a short duration of action. The dose should be limited to 3 mg kg⁻¹ of local anaesthetic (0.06 g kg⁻¹ of cream) because uptake across mucous membranes is rapid. EMLA is not licensed for dental anaesthesia in the UK.

### Anaesthesia of wounds

EMLA can be repeatedly applied to minor wounds (e.g. circumcision) to provide postoperative pain relief. No complications have been reported, but uptake of local anaesthetic across open wounds has not been measured and EMLA is not recommended for this use in the UK.

## Contraindications

### Concurrent treatment with methaemoglobin-inducing agents (e.g. sulphonamides, primaquine, nitrates, phenacetin)

Methaemoglobin-inducing agents oxidize haemoglobin at a greater rate than the red blood cells' ability to reduce methaemoglobin. The absorption of prilocaine will compound this effect. Serious methaemoglobinaemia has occurred when EMLA was applied to the skin of a 12-week-old baby taking trimethoprim-sulphamethoxazole (co-trimoxazole).

### Congenital or idiopathic methaemoglobinaemia

Prilocaine is a known inducer of methaemoglobin.

### Sensitivity to amide local anaesthetics

Genuine sensitivity to amide anaesthetics is extremely rare and is usually associated with chronic application of perianal preparations.

### Open wounds

Absorption across wounds has not been measured and EMLA is not yet recommended for application to surgical incisions (see above).

### Immature skin

Unfortunately EMLA is not licensed in the UK for use in children under 12 months of age, although it has been shown to be safe in normal babies older than 3 months in a dose of 2 g applied to 16 cm² of skin for less than 4 hours. Younger babies, particularly premature babies, have very permeable skin and potential for significant absorption of local anaesthetics.

*Eczema and dermatitis*

Local anaesthetics are more rapidly absorbed across diseased skin. Plasma concentrations of lignocaine and prilocaine associated with the application of EMLA to areas of eczema or dermatitis have not been measured and use of EMLA is not recommended in these conditions.

## Complications

### Hypersensitivity

Hypersensitivity to amide local anaesthetics is extremely rare (see above) and has not been reported for EMLA.

### Systemic toxicity and anaesthesia of the upper airway

Anaesthesia of the upper airway and probable systemic toxicity has been reported in children who have licked EMLA from the site of application.

## FURTHER READING

Freeman, J. A., Doyle, E., Tee Im, N. G., and Morton, N. S. (1993). Topical anaesthesia of the skin: a review. *Paediatric Anaesthesia*, **3**, 129–38.

Gajraj, N. M., Pennant, J. H., and Watcha, M.F. (1994). Eutectic mixture of local anaesthetics (EMLA®) cream. *Anesthesia Analgesia*, **78**, 574–83.

Woolfson, D., and McCafferty, D. (1993). *Percutaneous local anaesthesia*. Ellis Horwood, New York.

## REFERENCES

### General

Bjerring, P., and Arendt- Nielsen, L. (1990). Depth and duration of skin analgesia to needle insertion after topical application of EMLA cream. *British Journal of Anaesthesia*, **64**, 173–7.

Engberg, G., Danielson, K., Henneberg, S., and Nilsson, A. (1987). Plasma concentrations of prilocaine and lidocaine and methaemoglobin formation in infants after epicutaneous application of a 5% lidocaine–prilocaine cream (EMLA). *Acta Anaesthesiologica Scandinavica.* **31**, 624–8.

Frayling, I. M., Addison, G. M., Chattergee, K., and Meakin, G. (1990). Methaemoglobinaemia in children treated with prilocaine–lignocaine cream. *British Medical Journal*, **301**, 153–4.

Jakobson, B. and Nilsson, A. (1985). Methemoglobinemia associated with a prilocaine–lidocaine cream and trimethoprim-sulphamethoxazole. A case report. *Acta Anaesthesiologica Scandinavica*, **29**, 453–5.

James, I. G. (1990). EMLA: complications. *British Journal of Anaesthesia*, **65**, 295.

Norman, J. and Jones, P. L. (1990). Complications of the use of EMLA. *British Journal of Anaesthesia*, **64**, 403.

## Clinical applications

Ashinoff, R. and Geronemus, R. G. (1990). Effect of the topical anesthetic EMLA on the efficacy of pulsed dye laser treatment of port-wine stain. *Journal of Dermatologic Surgery and Oncology*, **16**, 1008–11.

Haasio, J., Jokinen, T., Numminen, M., and Rosenberg, P. H. (1990). Topical anaesthesia of gingival mucosa by 5% eutectic mixture of lignocaine and prilocaine or by 10% lignocaine spray. *British Journal of Oral and Maxillofacial Surgery*, **28**, 99–101.

Hallén, B. and Uppfeldt, A. (1982). Does lidocaine–prilocaine cream permit painfree insertion of IV catheters in children? *Anesthesiology*, **57**, 340–2.

Hallén, B., Olsson, G. L., and Uppfeldt, A. (1984). Pain-free venepuncture. *Anaesthesia*, **39**, 969–72.

Halperin, D., *et al.* (1989). Topical skin anesthesia for venous, subcutaneous drug reservoir and lumbar punctures in children. *Pediatrics*, **84**, 281–4.

Hopkins, C. S., Buckley, C. J., and Bush, G. H. (1988). Pain-free injection in infants. *Anaesthesia*, **43**, 198–201.

MacKinlay, G. A. (1988). Save the prepuce. Painless separation of preputial adhesions in the outpatient clinic. *British Medical Journal*, **297**, 590–1.

Maunuksela, E. L. and Korpela, R. (1986). Double-blind evaluation of a lignocaine–prilocaine cream (EMLA) in children. *British Journal of Anaesthesia*, **58**, 1242–5.

Miser, A. W. *et al.* (1994). Trial of a topically administered local anaesthetic (EMLA cream) for pain relief during central venous port accesses in children with cancer. *Journal of Pain Symptom Management*, **9**, 259–64.

Ogborn, M.R. (1992). The use of a eutectic mixture of local anesthetic in pediatric renal biopsy. *Pediatric Nephrology*, **6**, 276–7.

Rosdahl, I., Edmar, B., Gisslén, H., Nordin, P., and Lillieborg, S. (1988). Curettage of molluscum contagiosum in children: analgesia by topical application of a lidocaine/prilocaine cream (EMLA®). *Acta Dermato-Venereologica*, **68**, 149–53.

Sirimanna, K. S., Madden, G. J., and Miles, M. B. (1990). Anaesthesia of the tympanic membrane: comparison of EMLA cream and iontophoresis. *Journal of Laryngology Otology*, **104**, 195–6.

Small, J., Wallace, R. G., Millar, R., Woolfson, A. D., and McCafferty, D. F. (1988). Pain-free cutting of split skin grafts by application of a percutaneous local anaesthetic cream. *British Journal of Plastic Surgery*, **41**, 539–43.

Smith, M., Gray, B. M., Ingram, S., and Jewkes, D. A. (1990). Double-blind comparison of topical lignocaine–prilocaine cream (EMLA) and lignocaine infiltration for arterial cannulation in adults. *British Journal of Anaesthesia*, **65**, 240–2.

Soliman, I. E., Broadman, L. M., Hannallah, R. S., and McGill, W. A. (1988). Comparison of the analgesic effects of EMLA (Eutectic Mixture of Local Anesthetics) to intradermal lidocaine infiltration prior to venous cannulation in unpremedicated children. *Anesthesiology*, **68**, 804–6.

Svensson, P. and Petersen, J. K. (1992). Anesthetic effect of EMLA occluded with orahesive oral bandages on oral mucosa. A placebo-controlled study. *Anesthesia Progress*, **39**, 79–82.

Watson, A. R., Szymkiw, P., and Morgan, A. G. (1988). Topical anaesthesia for fistula cannulation in haemodialysis patients. *Nephrology, Dialysis and Transplantation*, **3**, 800–802.

## Lignocaine

Lignocaine is available either as a hydrochloride salt in a solution (0.5, 1, 2 or 4 per cent) or gel (2 per cent), or as a formulation of the unionized base either as an ointment (5 per cent) or 10 per cent solution in alcohol. Lignocaine in these formulations penetrates intact skin poorly but is rapidly absorbed across mucous membranes. Absorption of lignocaine across intact skin from an aqueous gel can be improved by adding an absorption promoter (e.g. glycyrrhetinic acid monohemiphthalate disodium).

### Indications

#### Dental anaesthesia

Lignocaine gel (2 per cent) or ointment (5 per cent) can be applied to the oral mucosa for 2–3 minutes to provide analgesia before dental block. The preparation can be held in place on the oral mucosa with a dental roll.

*Fibre-optic intubation in awake children*
The technique of fibre-optic intubation is occasionally used in awake babies and children. Solutions of lignocaine HCl can be used to provide surface anaesthesia. The dose should be limited to 3 mg kg$^{-1}$ to reduce the risk of toxic reactions.

*Anaesthesia of wounds*
Lignocaine (e.g. 2 per cent, 5 per cent ointment, 10 per cent spray) can be applied to provide excellent analgesia after minor operations, e.g. circumcision. The technique is simple and parents can re-apply local anaesthetic to provide prolonged analgesia after discharge from hospital. There are no reported complications but the uptake of local anaesthetic across wounds has been measured only in a small number of boys having circumcision. The safety of the technique, particularly if local anaesthetic is re-applied, has not been adequately assessed.

## Contraindications

(1)  Sensitivity to amide local anaesthetics;
(2)  (relative contraindication) application to wounds.

## REFERENCES

Andersen, K. H. (1989) A new method of analgesia for relief of circumcision pain. *Anaesthesia*, **44**, 118–20.

Kano, T., Hashiguchi, A., Nakamura, M., Morioka, T., Mishumi, M., and Nakano, M. (1992). A comparative study of transdermal 10% lidocaine gel with and without glycyrrhetinic acid monohemiphthalate disodium for pain reduction at venous cannulation. *Anesthesia Analgesia*, **74**, 535–8.

Tree-Trakarn, T. and Pirayavaraporn, S. (1985). Postoperative pain relief for circumcision in children: comparison among morphine, nerve block, and topical analgesia. *Anesthesiology*, **62**, 519–22.

Tree-Trakarn, T., Pirayavaraporn, S., and Lertakyamanee, J. (1987). Topical analgesia for relief of post-circumcision pain. *Anesthesiology*, **67**, 395–9.

## Adrenaline–cocaine mixture

A liquid or gel mixture containing adrenaline 1 : 2000 and cocaine 11.8 per cent, with or without tetracaine (amethocaine)

0.5 per cent, can be applied to minor wounds and is used in North America to provide anaesthesia for debridement or suturing. These mixtures produce analgesia comparable to intradermal infiltration with lignocaine but with greater patient compliance. They are more effective for proximal than distal lacerations. Adrenaline–cocaine mixtures should be applied until the wound blanches (approximately 20–30 minutes).

The components of adrenaline–cocaine mixtures are potent and present in high concentrations. There is no published maximum safe dose.

## Contraindications

### Application to extensive burns or mucous membranes
Amethocaine and cocaine are absorbed rapidly across mucous membranes and burnt skin and may produce systemic toxicity.

### Application to poorly vascularized areas
Cocaine and adrenaline are vasoconstrictors and should not be applied to parts of the body supplied by end arteries (e.g. the penis and digits) or with a poor blood supply (e.g. the pinna of the ear and tip of the nose) because of the risk of gangrene.

## Complications

### Systemic toxicity
Systemic toxicity (including convulsions, disorientation, hallucinations, and death) can occur if adrenaline–cocaine mixtures are ingested or applied to mucous membranes, burns, or extensive lacerations.

### Gangrene
Skin necrosis can occur if adrenaline–cocaine mixtures are applied to areas with a poor blood supply.

## REFERENCES

Anderson, A. B., Colecchi, C., Baronski, R., DeWitt, T. G. (1990). Local anesthesia in pediatric patients: topical TAC versus lidocaine. *Annals of Emergency Medicine*, **19**, 519–22.

Bonadio, W. A. and Wagner, V. R. (1992). Adrenaline–cocaine gel topical anesthetic for dermal laceration repair in children. *Annals of Emergency Medicine*, **21**, 1435–7.

Hegenbarth, M. A., *et al.* (1990). Comparison of topical tetracaine, adrenaline, and cocaine anesthesia infiltration for repair of lacerations in children. *Annals of Emergency Medicine*, **19**, 63–7.

Tipton, G. A., DeWitt, G., and Eisenstein, S. J. (1989). Topical TAC (tetracaine, adrenaline, cocaine) solution for local anesthesia in children: prescribing inconsistency and acute toxicity. *Southern Medical Journal*, **82**, 1344–6.

# 4

## *Wound instillation and infiltration*

S. J. MATHER

### Indications

Wound infiltration and 'field block' are very commonly used in paediatric anaesthesia, particularly if a regional technique has not been employed. Local anaesthetic agents can be injected pre- or postoperatively by the anaesthetist or the surgeon. Additionally, solution can be instilled into open wounds before closure, when the local anaesthetic will 'fix' on to the tissues.

Infiltration is particularly useful after pyloromyotomy, hernia repair, and in most superficial wounds.

### Contraindication

Local infection

### Equipment for infiltration

A 25 g 3.5 cm (retrobulbar) needle is especially suitable for field block where all sites of the proposed incision can usually be infiltrated from one or two skin punctures. For most wounds, however, a standard 23 g intramuscular needle is acceptable.

### Drugs

Lignocaine (up to 6 mg kg$^{-1}$) with adrenaline, or bupivacaine (up to 2.5 mg kg$^{-1}$) with or without adrenaline. Care must be taken to avoid toxic limits as large volumes of solution may be required. The doses (mg per kg) quoted may be diluted to the volume needed to perform the infiltration. For example, if the maximum dose of bupivacaine in a 10 kg child is 25 mg (10 ml of 0.25 per cent solution), this may be diluted to give, say, 25 ml for infiltration of a large incision or several smaller wounds. It must be

remembered that lignocaine has a shorter onset time than bupivacaine and is therefore more suitable for preoperative use unless
sufficient time is given for the bupivacaine to act. If the infiltration
is an accompaniment to general anaesthesia, as is usually the case,
bupivacaine is the preferred agent as it will provide longer-lasting
postoperative analgesia.

### Technique

The use of small needles (27 g) and warmed local anaesthetic solution minimizes discomfort on injection in the conscious child.

Clean surgical wounds may be infiltrated from the cut edges
without puncturing the skin.

Lacerations may already be contaminated by bacteria, which
may spread along the needle track.

If field block is being performed, one should aim to deposit the
solution so as to surround the lesion to be excised. It is advisable
to infiltrate both skin and muscle layers. If the needle tip is kept
moving, the risk of inadvertent intravascular injection is small.

### Complications

(1)  Inadvertent intravascular injection;
(2)  haematoma;
(3)  local anaesthetic toxicity.

## REFERENCES

Davidson, J. A. and Boom, S. J. (1992). Warming lignocaine to reduce
    pain associated with injection. *British Medical Journal*, **305**, 617–18.
Jöhr, M., Hess, F. A., and Gerber, H. (1994). Warming and alkalinisa-
    tion of lidocaine equally reduce pain associated with injection.
    *Anesthesia Analgesia*, **78**, S180.
McNicol, L. R., Martin, C. S., Smart, N. G., and Logan, R. W. (1990).
    Peroperative bupivacaine for pyloromyotomy pain. *Lancet*, **1**, 54–5.
Sury, M. R. J., McLuckie, A., and Booker, P. D. (1990). Local analgesia
    for infant pyloromyotomy. Does wound infiltration with bupivacaine
    affect postoperative behaviour? *Annals of The Royal College of Surgeons
    of England*, **72**, 324–8.

# Part 3

# Techniques of regional anaesthesia: nerve blockade

# 5

# *Nerve blocks for dental surgery*

## I. BALL

## INTRODUCTION

A careful painless injection technique is one of the most important aspects of administering dental local analgesia to children because, unlike adults, it is rare that a hurt child who becomes frightened and distraught will allow one to continue with treatment, let alone permit a second attempt at such an injection. Equally important is a simple straightforward explanation to the child to reassure him or her about the procedure, avoiding reference to frightening or emotive words such as needle or injection. It is usually sufficient to tell the child that the tooth and face will 'go to sleep but wake up later'. Because of the disconcerting sensation it is also good practice to reassure the child by showing him with the aid of a mirror that although his face feels different his appearance remains unaltered.

Unlike most local analgesic techniques described in this book which are performed under light general anaesthesia, local analgesia in dentistry is frequently used alone even in small children. The syringe should never be prepared for use in front of the child and he or she should never be allowed to see the unsheathed hypodermic needle. Surface analgesic cream or gel, such as lignocaine gel, should be used prior to the injection and sufficient time allowed for it to become effective. The syringe should be kept out of the child's line of vision.

An important principle when giving these injections in a sensitive area like the mouth, is slowly to inject a small quantity of analgesic solution ahead of the advancing needle tip. This not only anaesthetises the tissue ahead of the needle which thereby reduces discomfort, but also allows the ball of solution at the

needle tip to displace nerves and blood vessels out of its advancing path and thus reduce the likelihood of damage to these
structures.

### Difficulties (Pulpal versus periodontal analgesia)

Most injections are usually given to achieve pulpal analgesia to
carry out dental restorations. With the possible exception of the
inferior alveolar nerve block, no single injection will render both
buccal and palatal gingivae and periodontium sufficiently analgesic to perform dental extractions, and thus palatal or lingual
injections (Fig. 5.10) are required in addition to buccal injections
to undertake such treatment.

### General complications of dental blocks

(1)  pain on injection;
(2)  inadvertent intravascular injection (minimized by using an
     aspirating syringe);
(3)  soft tissue damage (minimized by meticulous technique);
(4)  'lip biting' in small children (caution parents);
(5)  haematoma in bleeding disorders and where the needle
     penetrates a venous plexus.


## INFILTRATION ANALGESIA

This is the simplest and most frequently used technique for
administering local analgesia to a child. It involves depositing the
solution submucosally next to the periosteum as close as possible
to the desired site or tooth to be anaesthetized, when it will
diffuse through the neighbouring soft tissues and cortical bone to
block all pain fibres in the vicinity.

Dental infiltration analgesia is generally more reliable, rapid,
and effective in children than in adults because the cortical plate
and supporting cancellous bone of the alveolus is less dense and
therefore more permeable than in adults, which facilitates per-
meation of the solution to the apices of the teeth. Although the
infiltration technique is not normally effective for lower molars
because of the dense impermeable outer cortical plate in the
mandible, it can be used to anaesthetize lower molars in children
under about 7 years of age.

*Indications*

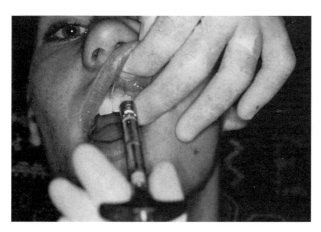

**Fig. 5.1** Infiltration analgesia is used for maxillary incisors, canines, and premolars, and the lower incisors (although injections into the labial sulcus adjacent to maxillary incisors may be painful). Surface analgesic cream should be applied prior to injection. The mucosa is drawn over the bevel of the needle. A small amount of solution is injected before advancing the needle tip approximately 1 cm until it is opposite the root apex when 1 ml should be injected with periodic aspiration.

Infiltration analgesia is applicable to virtually all the maxillary teeth: incisors, canines, premolars, and molars (Fig. 5.1). In the maxilla the nasal spine in the labial sulcus above the central incisors and the zygomatic buttress in the permanent first molar region limits the depth to which the needle can be inserted and the available tissue into which the fluid can diffuse. In the latter case the apices of this molar are deeply within the bone and are much higher and deeper than the reflection of the buccal sulcus. Injections in the labial sulcus adjacent to the maxillary incisors are notoriously painful unless done with great care (Fig. 5.1).

In the mandible, infiltration analgesia is mostly confined to the lower incisors (Fig. 5.2). A labial sulcus injection deposits the solution near the apices of these teeth where the cortical plate of bone is so thin and permeable that diffusion into the alveolus is almost instantaneous. Because of the increasing thickness of the compact cortical plate with age, infiltration for dental analgesia is inappropriate in the mandibular molar regions in children over the age of about 7 years and the inferior alveolar (dental) block is then called for (Fig. 5.5).

Infiltration injections are routinely used for soft-tissue analgesia.

## Equipment

1) A dental syringe such as the Astra Aspiject® suitable for use with self-aspirating dental cartridges.
2) Short (2.5 cm) 30 g hypodermic needle.

## Drugs

Self-aspirating 2.2 ml cartridges of either prilocaine hydrochloride 3 per cent EP (Citanest®) with 0.3 iu ml$^{-1}$ felypressin, or lignocaine hydrochloride 2 per cent (Xylocaine®) with 1 : 80 000 adrenaline.

If it is desired to shorten the duration of analgesia for the comfort of the patient, 4 per cent prilocaine (which has mild vasodilatory properties) may be used without a vasoconstrictor in children.

## Technique

The chair should be tilted backwards about 30–45° to improve access and visibility for the operator, and to avoid the child seeing the syringe.

The orientation of the tooth should be noted and the position of its apex assessed in relation to the buccal sulcus. In a child the distance of the root apex from the gum margin may be three or four times the height of the clinical crown.

Prior to the injection a small amount of surface analgesic cream should be applied to the pre-dried mucosa at the injection site using a cotton wool roll or a cotton bud and remain *in situ* for 2 minutes.

When the operator is ready to give the injection, the syringe should preferably be passed to and correctly orientated in the palm of the operator's hand by an assistant who remains at hand to comfort and, if necessary, gently restrain the child.

The cheek is held between the index finger and thumb of one hand, and the vestibular mucosa is stretched taught by pulling the cheek outwards. The needle tip is placed with its bevel towards the mucosa at the reflection of the buccal sulcus op-

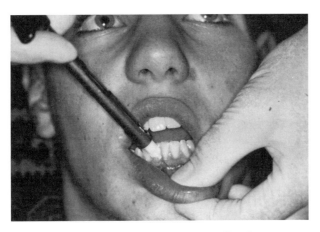

**Fig. 5.2**   Mandibular incisor infiltration.

posite the tooth to be anaesthetized and the taught mucosa is pulled gently over it. A small amount of solution is simultaneously expressed into the submucosal tissues. Holding the cheek in the manner described exerts firm yet gentle control over the child's face and prevents the child pulling away, or making sudden head movements during the injection procedure (Fig. 5.2).

The needle should be gradually advanced submucosally a centimetre or so, slowly injecting a small amount of solution ahead of the tip to anaesthetize the deeper tissues and reduce discomfort, until the needle tip is approximately opposite the root apex. About half a cartridge of local analgesic solution (1 ml) should be slowly injected at this site, periodically releasing the pressure on the handle of the self-aspirating syringe to check that the solution is not being injected intravascularly, and avoiding a forceful injection which would rapidly distend the tissues and cause pain.

The needle tip must remain supraperiosteally. Perforation of the periosteum and injection of the solution below it can strip it from the underlying bone and may cause severe postoperative pain. Ideally, the needle should not pass into muscle tissue nor should the solution be deposited there. Not only does this cause similar postoperative discomfort, but it also renders the analgesic solution less effective.

*Other infiltration injections*

To supplement an inferior alveolar nerve block a *long buccal nerve infiltration injection* is given submucosally 1 cm into the substance of the cheek opposite the mandibular retro-molar region where the vertical ramus joins the horizontal ramus of the jaw. That and a lingual sulcus injection (Fig. 5.10) between the tongue and the mandibular teeth are both occasionally useful to anaesthetize aberrant nerve branches that enter the body of the mandible through tiny foramina to supply the teeth from sources such as the long buccal branch of the trigeminal nerve or the cutaneous colli nerves from the neck.

## THE INTRALIGAMENTARY INJECTION

*Indications*

This technique is most valuable in children to achieve local analgesia of individual teeth without widespread loss of sensation of neighbouring soft tissues such as the lips and cheeks.

*Equipment*

A variety of special syringes (Peripress®, Citoject®, Jet inject®, Ligmaject®, for example) are available to administer local analgesic solution under high pressure into the periodontal membrane or ligament, between the bony wall of the socket and the tooth. These special syringes use an ultra-short (1.1 cm) 30 gauge hypodermic needle.

*Drugs*

Dental cartridges of lignocaine or prilocaine.

*Specific complications*

The technique does have some theoretical disadvantages, one being the implantation of oral bacteria deep into the socket, and another the possibility of ischaemic necrosis of the periodontal tissues resulting from the action of the vasoconstrictor in the local anaesthetic solution and the extreme pressure needed to inject the solution. Flooding the periodontal membrane with analgesic solution in this way may cause slight extrusion of the tooth from its socket and it has also been suggested that the solution itself may exert a toxic effect on the developing permanent tooth germ below the primary tooth being treated, although this is unsubstantiated.

## Technique

The technique involves the use of an ultra-short 30 gauge hypodermic needle which is inserted into the gingival sulcus at the neck of the tooth alongside first the mesial and then the distal papillae angled at approximately 30° to the long axis of the root and gently advanced down the socket wall while continuously expressing the solution under pressure into the periodontal membrane (Fig. 5.3).

The extreme back pressure which develops within the cartridge as local analgesic solution is forced into the periodontal space can cause

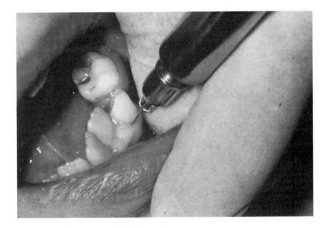

**Fig. 5.3**   Intraligamentary injection. This technique can be used to produce analgesia of individual teeth very rapidly. It avoids numbness in the surrounding soft tissues which is advantageous. A special high-pressure syringe and ultra-short needle are required. The needle is inserted into the gingival sulcus at the neck of the tooth alongside first the mesial then distal papillae, angled at 30° to the long axis of the root. Analgesic solution is expressed as the needle is advanced down the socket wall. Onset of analgesia is extremely rapid.

the glass to shatter and this is why the cartridge must always be protected by a tubular plastic sheath inside the body of the syringe.

Because all teeth in young children are constantly re-adjusting to a new occlusion, the periodontal membrane is in a perpetual state of reorganization and therefore has a liberal blood supply and is many times wider than it is in adults. This facilitates insertion of the needle and makes the technique relatively simple to administer.

Analgesia is instantaneous and it is frequently possible to pick up the forceps and extract the tooth immediately after putting down the syringe!

With care the technique can be administered virtually painlessly in children and because it does not 'numb' large areas of the face, lips, and cheeks, there is less likelihood of the child biting himself before normal sensation returns (Fig. 5.4).

## REGIONAL NERVE BLOCK INJECTIONS

From an anaesthetist's viewpoint these are the most important local analgesic techniques used in children's dentistry. They comprise the inferior alveolar nerve block, the mental nerve block, the infraorbital nerve block, the posterior superior alveolar nerve block (otherwise known as the maxillary molar nerve block), also

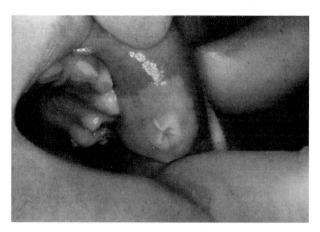

**Fig. 5.4** Mucosal damage due to biting a numb lip. Soft-tissue damage such as this can be minimized by the intraligamentary technique, which does not anaesthetize the surrounding soft tissues.

the anterior palatal nasopalatine nerve block and the posterior palatal greater palatine nerve block.

## *Indications*

These effectively anaesthetize not only the teeth but large sections of the oral mucosae and the skin of the face and are useful for performing surgery in situations where general anaesthesia may not be possible or where the patient can be only lightly sedated.

## *Equipment*

As for infiltration analgesia, but in older children a 'long' 27 gauge hypodermic needle (3.0 cm) may be required for inferior alveolar nerve blocks.

## *Drugs*

As for infiltration analgesia.

In general, the most appropriate way of embarking upon a regional nerve block is to palpate the bony landmarks of the skull in the location associated with the emergence of the nerve from, or entry into, its bony canal.

## Inferior alveolar nerve block

The most difficult regional block to perform is the inferior alveolar nerve block, because it involves a long path of insertion of the needle and it is difficult to visualize where the needle is passing in relation to surrounding structures (Fig. 5.5a,b). The nerve is blocked where it enters through the mandibular foramen.

## *Indirect technique*

This requires that the operator should face the patient and with the patient's mouth widely open palpate the anterior border of the vertical ramus, both the internal and external oblique ridges, by placing the thumb horizontally along the occlusal surfaces of the lower teeth. Then, using the index finger of the same hand locate the posterior border of the mandible extra-orally just below the ear (the angle of the mandible can be detected extra-orally with the middle finger).

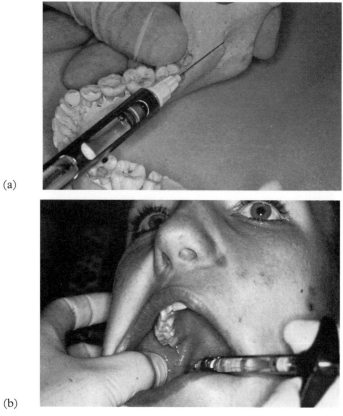

(a)

(b)

**Fig. 5.5** (a) Needle position for inferior alveolar block shown on a dry skull. The mandible is grasped with the finger and thumb. This photograph clearly shows the needle position in relation to the mandibular foramen. (b) Inferior alveolar nerve block. The operator faces the patient and with the mouth widely open palpates the anterior border of the vertical ramus of the mandible, both the anterior and posterior oblique ridges, by placing the thumb horizontally along the occlusal surfaces of the lower teeth. The index finger of the same hand is then used to locate the posterior border of the mandible extraorally just below the ear. This gives the operator an impression of the width of the vertical ramus. The needle is inserted just lateral to the pterygomandibular raphe alongside the internal oblique ridge and parallel with the thumb, then advanced 1–1.5 cm along the inner aspect of the mandible. The barrel of the syringe is then swung across to the opposite side of the jaw in the same horizontal plane. The needle is then further advanced until it strikes bone. It is withdrawn 1 mm or so and 1–2 ml of solution injected.

This enables the operator to gauge by proprioception between these two reference points the full anteroposterior width of the vertical ramus.

The mandibular foramen lies at the lingula approximately half-way between these two landmarks on a horizontal line on the inner aspect of the vertical ramus, and in children of school age, on a level with the occlusal plane of the mandibular teeth, or in pre-school children slightly below this level, i.e. parallel to and on a line with the gingival margins of the teeth.

The point of the needle is inserted through the mucosa just lateral to the pterygomandibular raphe alongside the internal oblique ridge and parallel with the thumb, and then advanced for approximately 1–1.5 cm along the inner aspect of the mandible.

The handle of the syringe is then swung across to the premolar region of the opposite side of the jaw and, while maintaining the same horizontal plane, advanced a further 1–1.5 cm, when the needle tip will strike bone in the vicinity of the lingula. The syringe should be withdrawn a fraction and 1–2 ml of solution deposited at this site.

This technique gives the added advantage that it allows the operator to grasp the child's jaw and thereby control head movements with one hand while holding the syringe in the other.

### Direct technique

This is the same as the indirect technique described above except that the syringe is angled so as to direct the needle tip at the lingula by placing the barrel of the syringe over the premolar teeth on the opposite side of the jaw from the outset.

## Mental nerve block

The mental nerve emerges below and between the root apices of the first and second mandibular premolars (in a young child the first and second primary molars).

### Equipment

As for infiltration analgesia.

## Drugs

As for infiltration analgesia.

## Technique

The technique essentially comprises an infiltration injection in the sulcus region at this site. It anaesthetizes the soft tissues of the lower lip up to the mid-line, and in children will also give buccal and pulpal analgesia to the teeth neighbouring the injection site. It will not usually anaesthetize lower incisors.

# Infraorbital nerve block

## Indication

This block is an invaluable technique to anaesthetize the upper lip and side of the face as well as the maxillary incisors, canine, and premolars.

## Equipment

As for infiltration analgesia.

## Drugs

As for infiltration analgesia.

## Technique

The inferior border of the infraorbital ridge is palpated using the index finger and its mid-point located. The tip of the index finger is then slid down into the bony depression 1 cm below this position on to the face to identify the site of the infraorbital foramen.

With the index finger maintained in this position, the upper lip is lifted with the thumb and an infiltration injection placed in the labial sulcus opposite the first premolar, or the first primary molar in a young child (Fig. 5.6).

Analgesic solution is continuously injected very slowly as the needle tip is advanced about 1 or 2 cm towards and deep to the index finger.

The depth of penetration of the needle depends on how far the sulcus can be extended by thumb pressure, as the position of the inferior orbital nerve is quite close to the buccal sulcus. The best means of assessing the correct position of the needle tip is by

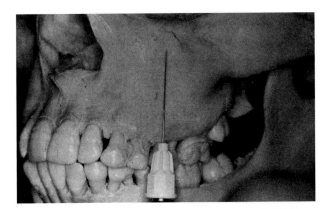

(a)

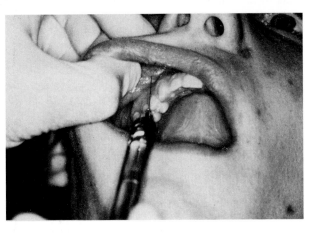

(b)

**Fig. 5.6**   Infraorbital nerve block. (a) The photograph shows the needle position for infraorbital nerve block on the dry skull of a 9-year-old child. (b) The inferior border of the infraorbital ridge is palpated extra-orally using the index finger to locate the mid-point. The finger is then slid into the bony depression 1 cm below this point, the site of the infraorbital foramen. The finger maintains this position while the upper lip is retracted with the thumb. An infiltration injection is placed in the labial sulcus opposite the first premolar (or the first primary molar in a young child). Solution is injected very slowly as the needle is gently advanced toward the infraorbital foramen, deep to the index finger. A bulge of analgesic solution should be felt by the palpating index finger when the needle tip is in the correct position. Gentle pressure with the finger frequently forces solution into the infraorbital canal, effecting profound analgesia of the incisor teeth and side of the face.

observing the swelling of local analgesic solution beneath the palpating index finger. Gentle pressure applied by the index finger will help spread the solution and often this will pass into the entrance of the infraorbital canal and effect profound analgesia of the side of the face and incisor teeth within 2 or 3 minutes.

## The posterior superior alveolar nerve block (maxillary molar nerve block)

### *Indication*
Analgesia of the pulps of the maxillary molars and premolars and the buccal gingiva.

### *Equipment*
As for infiltration analgesia.

### *Drugs*
As for infiltration analgesia.

### *Complications*
The older technique of blocking the posterior superior alveolar nerve has been associated with complications arising from inadvertent damage to the nearby pterygoid venous plexus, resulting in a substantial haematoma within the pterygomaxillary (infratemporal) fossae. These complications are much less likely with the maxillary molar nerve block technique described below.

### *Technique*
The original technique has now been superseded by the more reliable and safer maxillary molar nerve block (Adatia 1976).

When the mouth is wide open the coronoid process obstructs access to the posterior region of the maxillary buccal sulcus, therefore the mouth should be closed slightly and the lower jaw deviated to the injection side to allow the coronoid process to swing backwards, giving a better field of view.

The posterior border of the zygomatic process usually lies distal to the permanent first molar in a child and can be palpated in the buccal sulcus using the index finger.

Just as for a typical infiltration injection, the needle tip is placed at the full depth of the buccal sulcus a centimetre or so distal to the zygomatic buttress and the mucosa stretched by everting the cheek between index finger and thumb as previously described.

After penetrating the mucosa the needle tip is advanced about 1.5 cm *through the buccinator muscle* so that the solution can be deposited in the loose areolar tissue above it (Fig. 5.7). About 2 ml of solution is slowly injected at this site and observed to swell the sulcus mucosa which bulges downwards slightly.

The needle is withdrawn and the reservoir of solution massaged into the pterygomaxillary space by placing the index finger over the bulge and applying gentle pressure in an upward and medial direction.

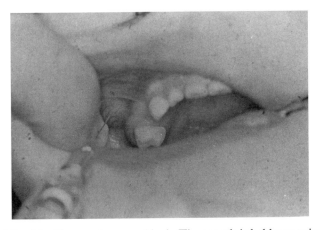

**Fig. 5.7** Maxillary molar nerve block. The mouth is held not quite fully open (to avoid obstruction by the coronoid process) and the lower jaw deviated to the injection side. The posterior border of the zygomatic process is palpated in the buccal sulcus distal to the permanent first molar. The needle is placed at the full depth of the buccal sulcus 1 cm distal to the zygomatic process. The needle is advanced 1.5 cm through the buccinator muscle and local analgesic solution injected into the loose areolar tissue above it. A 2 ml injection should produce a small bulge in the mucosa. The index finger is then used to massage this bulge and spread the solution into the pterygomaxillary space.

## Palatal infiltration injections

### Indication
Analgesia of the palatal mucosa adjacent to maxillary molars and premolars.

### Drugs
As for infiltration analgesia.

### Equipment
As for infiltration analgesia.

### Technique
These injections are best given in the thicker layer of the mucosa which lies midway between the gingival margins of the teeth and the palatal mid-line suture.

Use of surface analgesic cream is strongly recommended to reduce the pain of these injections.

The child should be psychologically prepared for the injection by telling him or her that they will feel a 'pinch' on the roof of the mouth and by demonstrating how this will feel by gently pinching the skin of the chin. If the child responds sensibly to this approach beforehand it is rare that he will remonstrate much during the procedure.

Allow the needle tip to touch the palatal mucosa while steadying the syringe against the other hand and gently express some solution as the tip is very gradually pressed against the surface. The needle should penetrate the mucosa to a depth of around 0.5 cm and be withdrawn slightly if it touches bone, when approximately 0.5 ml of solution may be injected (Fig. 5.8).

## The nasopalatine nerve block

### Indication
Analgesia of palatal mucosa adjacent to maxillary incisors and the anterior one-third of the palate.

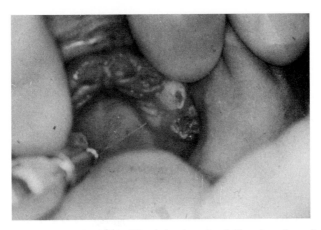

**Fig. 5.8** Palatal infiltration. The injection should be given into the thicker mucosa midway between the gingival margins of the teeth and the palatal mid-line suture. After the application of a liberal quantity of surface analgesic cream, the needle tip is placed against the mucosa and solution expressed as the tip is gently pressed against the surface. The needle is *very gradually* advanced through the mucosa to a depth of 0.5 cm and 0.5 ml of solution injected. The needle must be withdrawn slightly if bone contact is made.

## Equipment

As for infiltration analgesia.

## Drugs

As for infiltration analgesia.

## Technique

Unfortunately, this may be a very painful injection because the palatal mucosa is much more fibrous and therefore difficult to penetrate and cannot expand much to accommodate the analgesic solution.

The puncture is made palatal to the maxillary central incisors at the edge of the incisive papilla and the needle passed 4 or 5 mm into the tightly adherent mucosa before very slowly injecting about 0.2–0.5 ml of solution (Fig. 5.9).

*It is recommended that the needle does not enter the bony canal for fear of damaging nerves and blood vessels confined within it.*

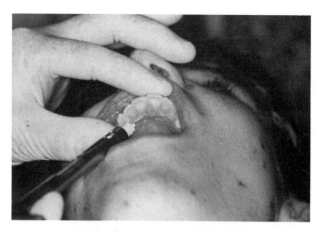

**Fig. 5.9** Nasopalatine nerve block. This injection may be painful due to the fibrous nature of the tissue. The needle is inserted palatal to the maxillary central incisors at the edge of the incisive papilla. The needle is advanced only 4 or 5 mm and then 0.2–0.5 ml solution is injected *very slowly. The needle should not enter the bony canal.*

## Greater palatine nerve block

### Indication

Analgesia of the posterior palatal mucosa, soft palate, and gingiva adjacent to the maxillary molars.

### Equipment

As for infiltration analgesia.

### Drugs

As for infiltration analgesia.

### Technique

0.2–0.5 ml of analgesic solution is injected 1 cm from the gingival margin approximately opposite the distal edge of the second maxillary molar with the needle as nearly at right angles to the surface of the mucosa as is possible.

This will block the greater palatine nerve as it emerges from the greater palatine canal.

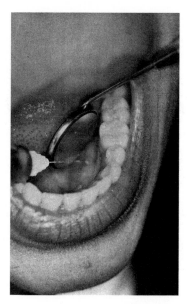

**Fig. 5.10**    Lingual (sulcus) infiltration analgesia.

## REFERENCES

Adatia, A. K. (1976). Regional nerve block for maxillary permanent molars. *British Dental Journal*, **140**, 87–92.

## FURTHER READING

Howe, G. L. and Whitehead, F. I. H. (1981). *Local anaesthesia in dentistry*, (23rd edn). Wright, Bristol.
Roberts, D. H. and Sowray, J. H. (1987). *Local analgesia in dentistry*, (3rd edn). Wright, Bristol.

# 6

## *Great auricular nerve block*

### S. J. MATHER

Apart from local infiltration and the dental blocks, the great auricular block is the only frequently performed block of the head and neck in children.

### Anatomy
The nerve pierces the fascia to become superficial over the sternomastoid muscle. Branches run up toward the mastoid process.

### Indications
Postoperative analgesia following mastoidectomy, tympanoplasty, or reduction of prominent ears (pinnaplasty).

### Contraindications
Local infection.

### Equipment
25 g 2.5 cm needle or dental cartridge syringe with 27 g needle.

### Drugs
2 per cent lignocaine or 0.25 per cent bupivacaine with adrenaline (1 : 80 000 adrenaline is often used with 2 per cent lignocaine to provide good vasoconstriction for tympanoplasty).

*Complications*

These are few and are largely as for infiltration analgesia. Inadvertent intravascular injection occurs rarely.

Subperiosteal injection may cause postoperative pain when the local anaesthetic wears off.

*Technique*

Two or three injections are made subcutaneously over the mastoid process (Fig. 6.1). Up to 10 ml may be required in an older child.

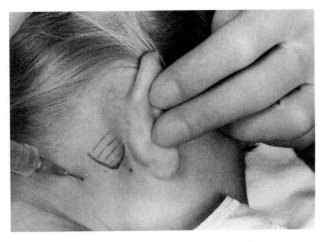

**Fig. 6.1**    Great auricular nerve block.

# 7

## *Upper limb blocks*

### S. J. MATHER

## BRACHIAL PLEXUS BLOCKS

### Introduction

These blocks, like most regional techniques in children, are usually used to supplement light general anaesthesia and more especially to provide good postoperative pain relief. Younger children are unlikely to tolerate the performance of anything other than wound infiltration without heavy sedation or general anaesthesia. Dalens, however, recommends brachial plexus blocks for emergency surgery on fractures of the arm in children with a possible full stomach. Axillary blocks alone are only really suitable for operations on the ulnar side of the forearm and hand as the musculo-cutaneous nerve is rarely blocked by this approach.

### Anatomy of the brachial plexus

The brachial plexus (Fig. 7.1) is formed by the ventral rami of C5, 6, 7, 8, and part of the ventral ramus of T1. Sometimes C4 and T2 make contributions to the plexus.

These nerves form the roots of the plexus which continues, with the subclavian artery, between the scalenus anterior and scalenus medius muscles, behind the mid-point of the clavicle and thence into the axilla, where the plexus exists as the lateral, medial and posterior cords. The branches of the plexus may be divided into supraclavicular and infraclavicular ones. The supraclavicular branches arise from the roots and trunks of the plexus (e.g. long thoracic nerve and suprascapular nerve) while the infraclavicular branches are derived from the cords and form the mixed nerves of the arm:

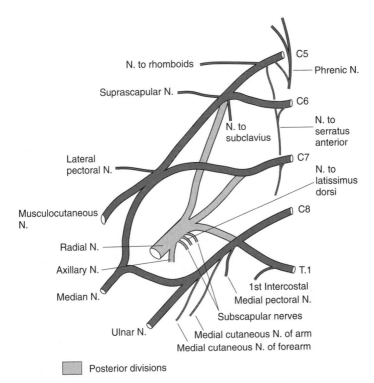

**Fig. 7.1** Plan of the brachial plexus. (N, nerve).

(1) lateral cord:
lateral pectoral C5, 6, 7,
musculocutaenous C5, 6, 7,
lateral root of median C5, 6, 7;
(2) medial cord:
medial pectoral C8, T1,
medial cutaneous of arm and forearm C8, T1,
ulnar C7, 8, T1,
medial root of median C8, T1;
(3) posterior cord:
upper subscapular C5, 6,
thoraco-dorsal C6, 7, 8,
lower subscapular C5, 6,
axillary C5, 6,
radial C5, 6, 7, 8, T1.

The supraclavicular and infraclavicular spaces are anatomically separated by fascial septa which also may limit the circumferential spread of analgesic solutions in the axillary space, resulting in incomplete block, particularly in areas supplied by the radial nerve (posterior cord) but also frequently those in the ulnar distribution.

### Equipment

Syringes of appropriate size for the dose. Short-bevelled 23 g stimulating needle, preferably insulated, with extension tube.

### Drugs

0.3 ml kg$^{-1}$ lignocaine 1 per cent or bupivacaine 0.25 per cent or occasionally 0.5 per cent plain solutions. Adrenaline-containing solutions reduce the rate of absorption but may be dangerous if injected intravascularly. There is a risk of intravascular injection, particularly with axillary brachial plexus blocks.

### Technique

Several approaches to the brachial plexus have been described:

|              |                      |
| ------------ | -------------------- |
| interscalene | (Winnie)             |
| parascalene  | (Dalens)             |
| subclavian   | (Winnie)             |
| supraclavicular | (Kulenkampff, Moore) |
| infraclavicular | (Raj)             |
| axillary     |                      |

Supraclavicular blocks are now rarely used and are probably contraindicated in children.

## Interscalene block (Winnie)

### Indications

Operations around the shoulder joint.

### Contraindications

Local infection, coagulopathy.

## Difficulties

The upper parts of the brachial plexus are easily blocked by this technique but the lower distributions are often missed, particularly the ulnar nerve.

## Complications

Phrenic nerve block is a major complication in a small infant due to greater dependence on diaphragmatic function. Recurrent laryngeal nerve block may also occur, as may block of the stellate ganglion, producing Horner's syndrome. There may be haematoma formation in the neck due to arterial or venous puncture. Spinal or epidural block may rarely occur.

## Technique

The patient is placed with the head at about 35° to the horizontal, turned away from the side to be blocked (Fig. 7.2). The point of insertion of the needle is located by reference to the cricoid cartilage. The interscalene space (which contains the roots, trunks, and part of the cords of the plexus) does not communicate with the neurovascular sheath in the axilla. Thus it follows that analgesic solution will not spread below the level of the coracoid process (where the two spaces are anatomically divided).

The Winnie interscalene technique seeks to inject local analgesic solution into the interscalene space at the level of C6 (cricoid cartilage). This minimizes danger to major vessels and avoids the pleura. A line drawn laterally from the cricoid cartilage passes over the tubercle of the transverse process of the sixth cervical vertebra (Chassaignac's tubercle) and crosses the interscalene groove which gives the point of needle puncture. A stimulating needle is inserted at 80° to the skin directed caudally and posteriorly (to avoid the vertebral artery and intervertebral foramen) towards the transverse process of the sixth cervical vertebra, which lies close to the skin. The needle should be advanced until twitches are elicited in the upper limb. If the bone of the transverse process is contacted before twitches are seen, a further attempt should be made with the needle angled more posteriorly.

## Parascalene block (Dalens)

### Indications

Operations around the shoulder joint.

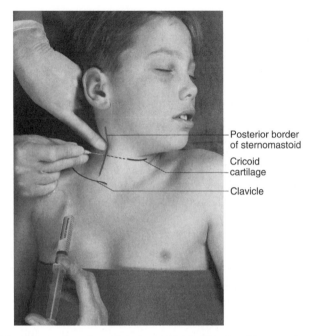

Posterior border
of sternomastoid

Cricoid
cartilage

Clavicle

**Fig. 7.2**   Interscalene brachial plexus block. The head is turned away
from the side to be blocked. The cricoid cartilage is marked and a line
drawn horizontally and laterally crosses the interscalene groove which
giving the point of needle puncture. A stimulating needle is inserted at
80° to the skin and is directed caudally and posteriorly, towards the
transverse process of C6. The needle is fixed when twitches are elicited
in the upper limb. If bone is contacted, further attempts should be made
with the needle directed more posteriorly.

*Contraindications*

Local infection, coagulopathy.

*Complications*

Vascular, and particularly arterial, puncture is rare with this technique, but the external jugular vein may be penetrated. This is
not usually a problem even in small infants. Horner's syndrome
occurs in less than 5 per cent of patients and phrenic nerve block
has not been reported.

*Technique*

This technique was developed to avoid major structures in the neck. The block was devised for use in children. Dalens *et al.* (1987) recommend that the child is laid supine with a rolled towel beneath the shoulders, the arm extended against the chest wall and the head turned to the opposite side (Fig. 7.3). As in the interscalene technique, the landmarks are found in relation to a line drawn between the cricoid cartilage and the transverse process of C6 (Chassaignac's tubercle), the line being drawn to the posterior edge of the sternomastoid muscle, and a further line from the mid-point of the clavicle to the transverse process of C6. The puncture is made at the junction of the upper two thirds and lower third of this line (Fig. 7.4).

An insulated stimulating needle is inserted at 90° to the skin and advanced posteriorly until twitches are seen. Dalens *et al.* (1987) recommended the injection of a small test dose following aspiration before the full dose is given. If the first attempt is unsuccessful at locating the nerve, the needle is reinserted slightly more laterally. This technique is usually successful in blocking both supraclavicular and infraclavicular branches of the plexus. According to Dalens the lower branches of the cervical plexus are also blocked in over 50 per cent of patients.

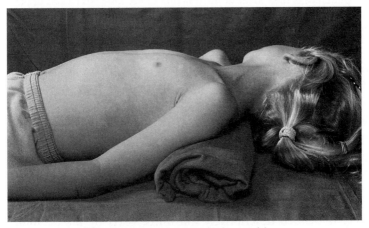

**Fig. 7.3** Parascalene block—position.

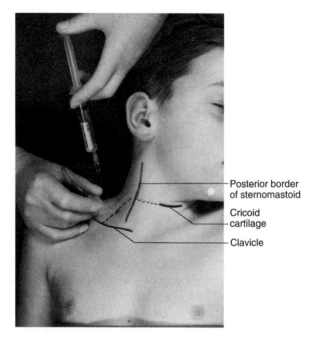

Posterior border
of sternomastoid

Cricoid
cartilage

Clavicle

**Fig. 7.4** Parascalene block. The child is placed in the supine position with a rolled towel beneath the shoulders, the arm extended against the chest wall, and the head turned to the opposite side. A line is then drawn between the cricoid cartilage and the tubercle of the transverse process of C6, as far as the posterior edge of the sternomastoid muscle. A further line is drawn from the mid-point of the clavicle to intersect the first line. The puncture is then made at the junction of the lower third and upper two-thirds of this line. A stimulating needle is inserted perpendicular to the skin and advanced until twitches are seen.

## Infraclavicular brachial plexus block (Raj infraclavicular block and axillary block)

### Anatomy

The brachial plexus is represented in the axilla by the three cords—lateral, posterior, and medial—which are closely related to the axillary artery. The nerves are sheathed with fascia which forms multiple compartments. This axillary space is not continuous with the interscalene space above the clavicle. The axillary artery is divided descriptively into three parts by the pectoralis minor muscle thus:

(1) first part—between the clavicle and the upper border of the muscle;
(2) second part—covered by the muscle itself; and
(3) third part—below the lower border of the muscle where the axillary artery becomes the brachial artery.

The cords of the brachial plexus give rise to the peripheral nerves in the lower part of the axilla. At the level of the third part of the axillary artery, the ulnar nerve lies medially, the radial posteriorly, and the median lateral to the artery. The musculocutaneous nerve and medial cutaneous nerve of the arm also lie in the axilla but are not closely related to the artery and are not usually blocked with the axillary approach.

### Indication

Infraclavicular blocks of the plexus are indicated for surgery on the forearm and hand, particularly to provide intra- and post-operative pain relief in conjunction with general anaesthesia. In the UK they are only very rarely used alone in children, but the axillary block may be useful in a co-operative older child if general anaesthesia is contraindicated. An axillary block is particularly suitable for postoperative pain relief after reduction of forearm fractures. Axillary block is by far the most common brachial block used and has a very low risk of significant complications.

### Contraindications

Local infection; coagulopathy.

### Equipment

A nerve stimulator and insulated needle are required for the Raj infraclavicular block. Short-bevelled 23 g or 25 g needles with extension tubes are sufficient for the axillary block. Long needles are sometimes required for obese patients. Use of a nerve stimulator to confirm close proximity to the nerve improves accuracy of placement but is an adjunct rather than a necessity for axillary blocks.

### Drugs

Lignocaine 1 per cent with adrenaline or bupivacaine 0.25 per cent (occasionally 0.5 per cent). A volume of 0.5 ml kg$^{-1}$ usually produces a good block. Bupivacaine 0.5 per cent may sometimes produce profound and long-lasting motor block in children, which may be distressing.

## Raj infraclavicular block

### Introduction

The Raj technique, although possibly safer than supraclavicular or subclavicular approaches above the axillary compartment, offers little advantage over axillary blocks and is difficult to perform in smaller children. The extent of the block is unpredictable due to variation in needle position and the speed and volume of the injection. If the musculocutaneous nerve remains unblocked, much of the theoretical advantage of the technique is lost.

### Technique

Raj's original paper (Raj *et al.* 1973) only describes the block in adults. The technique aims to block also the musculocutaneous nerve by entering the neurovascular sheath above the level at which the musculocutaneous nerve leaves the axilla. The infraclavicular approach avoids the great vessels of the neck and dome of the pleura. The extent of the block is very variable, depending upon spread of the local anaesthetic solution. The musculocutaneous nerve is not always blocked.

The patient is placed supine with the head turned to the opposite side and the arm abducted to (but not beyond) 90°. The landmarks (Figs 7.5, 7.6) are the mid-point of the clavicle, the axillary artery pulse in the axilla and the transverse process of C6, located as before. A line is then drawn from the transverse process of C6 to the point where pulsation of the axillary artery is felt. Dalens (1990) recommends simply drawing a line perpendicular to the mid-point of the clavicle. The site of needle insertion then lies on this line immediately lateral to the axillary artery (1–3 cm below the clavicle depending upon the size of the child). Using a nerve stimulator, an insulated short-bevelled needle with extension tube is inserted backward, slightly laterally, and slightly caudally until twitches are seen. The technique has been modified by Whiffler (1987) who recommends inserting the needle at right angles to the skin until twitches are seen. Whiffler, however, does not describe his technique (coracoid block) for use in children.

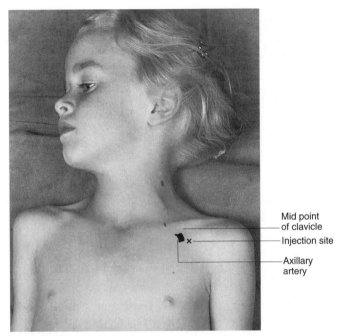

Mid point
of clavicle
Injection site
Axillary
artery

**Fig. 7.5**   The simplified landmarks for the infraclavicular block
(Dalens 1990) are the mid-point of the clavicle and the axillary artery.
The injection site is a point immediately lateral to the axillary artery on a
line perpendicular to the mid-point of the clavicle. The use of a nerve
stimulator is mandatory.

## Axillary brachial plexus block

Many axillary approaches have been described since the original
description by Hirschel in 1911. Due to the close relation of the
cords of the brachial plexus to the axillary artery, the neurovascular sheath can be located easily. Most authors seem to
favour locating the puncture site as high as possible in the axilla.
However, some favour a two-injection technique in order to
increase the likelihood of circumferential spread of the solution
around the artery and thus, hopefully, block all the nerves in the
sheath. Some anaesthetists prefer transfixion of the axillary artery
with the needle and then injecting local anaesthetic solution
behind and in front of the vessel. This technique, although much
used in adults without complications, should probably be avoided

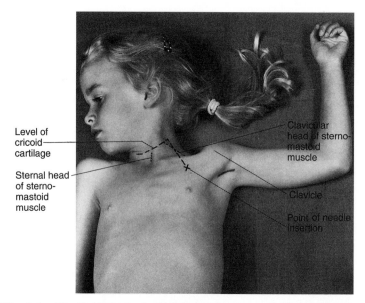

Level of
cricoid
cartilage

Sternal head
of sterno-
mastoid
muscle

Clavicular
head of sterno-
mastoid
muscle

Clavicle

Point of needle
insertion

**Fig. 7.6** The Raj infraclavicular block. The patient is placed supine with the arm abducted to 90°. The transverse process of C6 and the point of pulsation of the axillary artery in the axilla are joined by a line extended for a few centimetres below the clavicle. The point of needle insertion lies on this line immediately lateral to the axillary artery below the clavicle. An insulated stimulating needle is inserted slightly laterally and caudally from this point until twitches are seen. The use of a nerve stimulator is essential.

in children as haematoma formation may cause nerve compression, particularly after trauma to the limb. Some authors suggest the injection of large volumes of dilute local anaesthetic solution in an attempt to achieve greater spread. The benefit of this is limited, however, by the presence of numerous fascial septa around the nerves.

### Complications

These are extremely rare after axillary blocks. Haematoma formation or minor nerve damage occasionally occur.

## TECHNIQUES

### *Two-puncture technique*

After palpating the pulse, the needle is advanced at about 45° to the skin, pointing cephalad until the sheath is penetrated at the upper edge of the artery. Often a distinctive 'give' or 'click' is felt. The needle should be seen to pulsate distinctly (the position can be confirmed with the nerve stimulator) (Figs 7.7, 7.8). Half the dose is then deposited at the upper border of the artery. The needle is then withdrawn and reinserted into the sheath at the lower border of the artery and the remaining solution injected. Aspiration on the syringe should always be performed before injecting the dose.

### *Single-injection technique*

The artery is located high in the axilla and then compressed distally against the humerus by the finger (which also compresses the

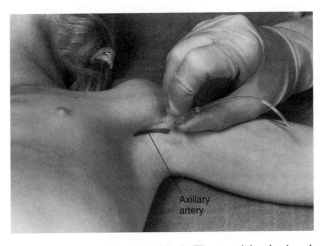

**Fig. 7.7**  Axillary brachial plexus block. The arterial pulse is palpated in the axilla and the skin marked. A sort-bevelled needle is advanced at 45° to the skin until a 'click' is felt. The needle should be seen to pulsate distinctly, and the position can be confirmed with a nerve stimulator if required. If a two-puncture technique is used, the needle is inserted at the upper border of the artery, where half the dose is given, and the manoeuvre repeated at the lower border.

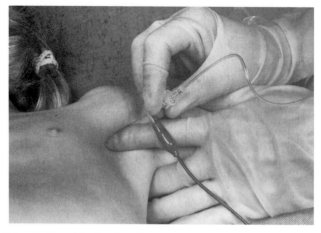

**Fig. 7.8**   Axillary block using the nerve stimulator. The artery is palpated as before. The needle is inserted high in the axilla and directed toward the artery. A 'click' should be felt as the sheath is penetrated. Using the nerve stimulator, twitches should be easily elicited with small stimulating currents. A single-injection technique suffices when the nerve stimulator is used to confirm accurate placement of the needle.

sheath, thus hopefully forcing the anaesthetic solution upwards and around the artery). The needle is inserted medially and cephalad until it enters the sheath where it should then pulsate (again, the position can be confirmed with the nerve stimulator). After careful aspiration without arterial compression, the full volume of solution is then given while the artery is again compressed. Compression should be maintained for a minute or two after injection in an attempt to spread the solution around the artery.

Both techniques, when successfully performed, result in good analgesia in the distribution of the ulnar and median nerves, but that in the radial distribution is less often complete. Occasionally the ulnar or median nerves remain unblocked. Supplementary nerve blocks at the wrist or elbow are then required. The musculocutaneous nerve is virtually never blocked by the axillary approach.

## REFERENCES

Dalens, B. J. (1990). Upper limb blocks. In *Paediatric regional anaesthesia*, (ed. B. J. Dalens). CRC Press, Boca Raton, Florida.

Dalens, B., Vanneuville, G., and Tanguy, A. (1987). A new parascalene approach to the brachial plexus in children: comparison with the supraclavicular approach. *Anesthesia Analgesia*, **66**, 1264–71.

Kulenkampff, D. and Persky, M. A. (1928). Brachial plexus anaesthesia: its indications, technic and dangers. *Annals of Surgery*, **87**, 883–91.

Moore, D. C. (1981). Supraclavicular approach for block of the brachial plexus. In *Regional block—a handbook for use in the clinical practice of medicine and surgery*, (ed. D. C. Moore), p. 221. Thomas, Springfield, Illinois.

Raj, P. P., Montgomery, S. J., Nettles, D., and Jenkins, M. T. (1973). Infraclavicular brachial plexus block—a new approach. *Anesthesia Analgesia*, **52**, 897–904.

Whiffler, K. (1987). Coracoid block—a safe and easy technique. *British Journal of Anaesthesia*, **53**, 845–8.

Williams, P. L., Warwick, R., Dyson, M., and Bannister, C. H. (1989). *Grays anatomy*, (37th edn). Churchill Livingstone, Edinburgh.

Winnie, A. P. (1970). Interscalene brachial plexus block. *Anesthesia Analgesia*, **49**, 455–66.

# NERVE BLOCK AT THE ELBOW

## Indication

These blocks may be used to supplement brachial plexus blocks.

## Contraindication

Local infection, coagulopathy.

## Median nerve

### Anatomy

The median nerve lies medial to the brachial artery in the ante-cubital fossa and runs between the biceps aponeurosis and then between the heads of the pronator teres muscle.

*Technique*

The injection is made on a line connecting the medial and lateral epicondyles of the humerus at a point just medial to the brachial artery (Figs 7.9, 7.10). The nerve should lie no more than 0.5 cm deep in a child. Up to 5 ml of local anaesthetic solution is injected, according to the size of the child.

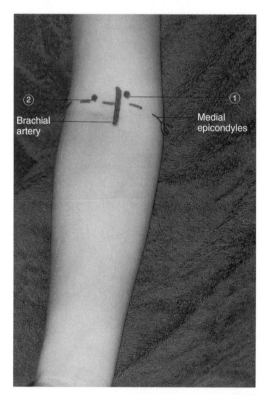

**Fig. 7.9**  Nerve block at the elbow. The medial and lateral epicondyles of the humerus are joined by a line drawn on the skin. The median nerve is blocked by an injection just medial to the brachial artery (1). The radial nerve and the lateral cutaneous nerve of the forearm are blocked by one injection (2): a short-bevelled needle is inserted between the brachioradialis muscle and the biceps tendon 1–2 cm lateral to the point where the biceps tendon crosses the intercondylar line. The needle is advanced toward the lateral epicondyle until bone contact is made. The injection is made as the needle is withdrawn. This manoeuvre is repeated twice with the needle more proximal each time.

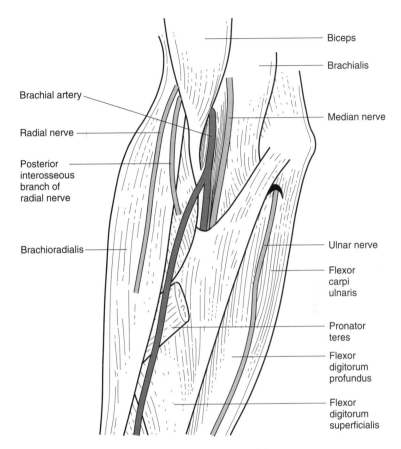

**Fig. 7.10** Anatomy of the elbow.

## Radial nerve and lateral cutaneous nerve of the forearm

The radial nerve can be blocked where it runs between the brachialis and brachioradialis muscles (Fig. 7.10). At the level of the head of the radius the nerve divides into deep and superficial branches. The lateral cutaneous nerve of the forearm runs on the lateral aspect of the biceps muscle proximal to the lateral epicondyle. Both nerves must be blocked to abolish cutaneous sensation along the radial side of the forearm.

### Technique

A line is drawn between the epicondyles. Both the radial nerve and lateral cutaneous nerve of the forearm can be blocked with one injection (Fig. 7.9). A short-bevelled needle is positioned between the brachioradialis muscle and the biceps tendon, 1–2 cm lateral to the point at which the biceps tendon crosses the intercondylar line. The needle is directed towards the most lateral point of the lateral epicondyle until bone contact is made. Local anaesthetic, 1–2 ml, is deposited as the needle is withdrawn off the bone. A further 2–4 ml are injected as the needle is almost fully withdrawn. The technique should then be repeated, working the needle tip more proximally until bone contact is made, so that two more 0.5–1 ml injections are made, each time after moving the needle more proximally up the lateral epicondyle.

## Ulnar nerve

Ulnar nerve block at the elbow is now less popular due to the possibility of ulnar neuritis following the block.

### Anatomy

The ulnar nerve is very superficial at the elbow and can be easily palpated against the bone where it lies between the medial epicondyle of the humerus and the olecranon.

### Technique

The arm must be flexed to 90° and internally rotated (Fig. 7.11). It can be placed conveniently across the chest. A short-bevelled needle is used, care being taken to avoid injection into the nerve. The needle is placed midway between the medial epicondyle and the olecranon and advanced distally. Up to 5 ml of local anaesthetic solution may be required, depending upon the age of the child. Intraneural block has been used (Löfstrom) but is not now recommended by most authors.

## REFERENCES

Löfstrom, B. (1969). In *Illustrated handbook in local anaesthesia*, (ed. E. Eriksson). Munksgaard 2300, Copenhagen S.

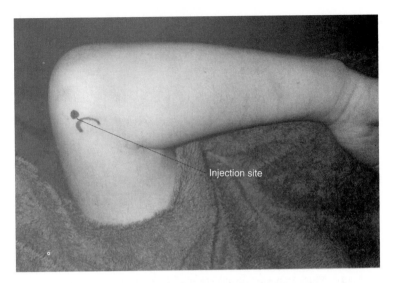

Injection site

**Fig. 7.11** Ulnar nerve block at the elbow. The ulnar nerve can be easily palpated in the groove between the medial epicondyle and the olecranon. The arm is flexed to 90° across the chest and a short-bevelled needle placed midway between the medial epicondyle and the olecranon and advanced distally. Up to 5 ml of solution is deposited, taking care to avoid injection into the nerve.

## WRIST BLOCK

*Indication*

This is used rarely in children but can be useful for postoperative analgesia following surgery on the hand. The median, ulnar and radial nerves are blocked in turn. Figure 7.12 shows the cutaneous distribution of the median radial and ulnar nerves in the hand.

*Contraindication*

Local infection.

### Median nerve

*Anatomy*

The nerve lies between the tendons of palmaris longus and flexor carpi radialis (Fig. 7.13).

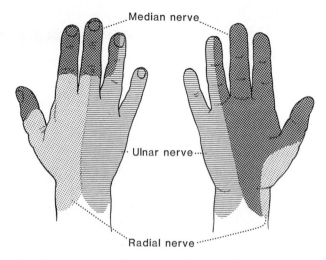

**Fig. 7.12** The cutaneous distribution of the median, radial and ulnar nerves at the wrist.

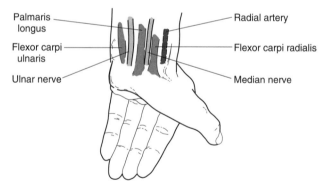

**Fig. 7.13** Anatomy of the wrist.

## Technique

The palmaris longus tendon (which is absent in some individuals) is identified. Immediately to the radial side of this tendon a short-

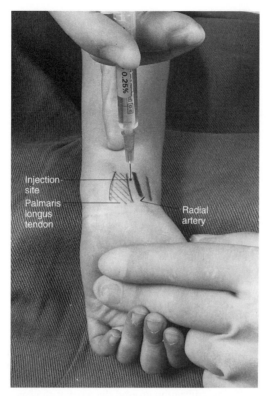

**Fig. 7.14**   Median nerve block at the wrist. The palmaris longus tendon is identified (if this is absent, a point medial to the flexor carpi radialis tendon is used). A short-bevelled needle is inserted immediately to the radial side of palmaris longus at the level of the ulnar styloid. A nerve stimulator can be used to elicit twitches in the thumb which confirms correct needle placement. Then 1–2 ml of local anaesthetic solution are injected.

bevelled needle is introduced to pierce the deep fascia at a point which is level with the ulnar styloid process (Fig. 7.14). Following confirmation of muscle twitching in the thumb using a nerve stimulator, 1–2 ml of local anaesthetic solution is injected. If the palmaris longus tendon is absent, a point medial to the flexor carpi radialis tendon is used instead.

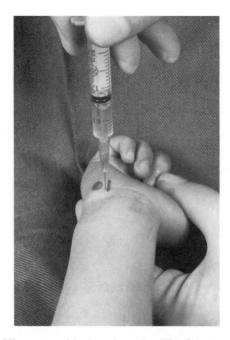

**Fig. 7.15**   Ulnar nerve block at the wrist. The flexor carpi ulnaris tendon is marked and a needle inserted between it and the ulnar artery at the level of the ulnar styloid. Accuracy can be improved by the use of a nerve stimulator. The dorsal cutaneous branch of the ulnar nerve is blocked by a half-ring infiltration around the wrist at the level of the ulnar styloid.

## Ulnar nerve

### Anatomy

The ulnar nerve lies in close relation to the lateral aspect of the flexor carpi ulnaris and deep to the ulnar artery.

### Technique

The nerve is blocked by passing a needle between the flexor carpi ulnaris tendon and the ulnar artery at the level of the ulnar styloid process (Fig. 7.15). Using a nerve stimulator to illicit twitches, 1–2 ml of local anaesthetic solution are then injected. The dorsal cutaneous branch is blocked by a half-ring infiltration around the wrist at the level of the ulnar styloid.

## Radial nerve block

### *Anatomy*

The radial nerve lies subcutaneously and supplies the dorsum of the hand on the radial side and the proximal parts of the dorsal aspect of the thumb, index, middle, and one-half of the ring finger.

### *Technique*

The nerve is easily blocked by a subcutaneous half-ring infiltration of local anaesthetic solution on the radial aspect of the wrist from a point lateral to the radial artery to the mid-point of the dorsum of the wrist, again at the level of the ulnar styloid (Fig 7.16). Dalens (1990) recommends that a line be drawn around the wrist at the level of the ulnar styloid process to facilitate all the components of the wrist block.

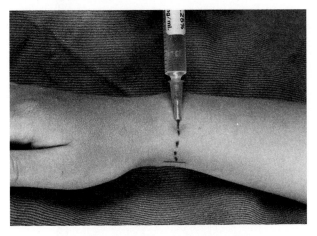

**Fig. 7.16** Radial nerve block at the wrist. The radial nerve is blocked by a subcutaneous half-ring infiltration from a point lateral to the radial artery to the mid-point of the dorsum of the wrist at the level of the ulnar styloid.

## REFERENCES

Dalens, B. J. (ed.) (1990). *Paediatric regional anaesthesia*, p. 268. CRC Press, Boca Raton, Florida.

Moore, D. C. (1981). Blocking the nerves of the arm at the elbow and wrist. In *Regional block. A handbook for use in the clinical practice of medicine and surgery*, (4th edn), (ed. D. C. Moore), p. 257. Charles C. Thomas, Springfield, Illinois.

Schulte-Steinberg, O. (1990). Blocks of the upper limb. In *Regional Anaesthesia in children*, (ed. C. St. Maurice and O. Schulte-Steinberg), p. 136. Appleton and Lange, Norwalk, Connecticut.

## DIGITAL NERVE BLOCKS—UPPER LIMB

### *Anatomy*

The dorsal aspects of the fingers are supplied by terminal branches of the radial and ulnar nerves, while the ventral aspects are supplied by the median and ulnar nerves.

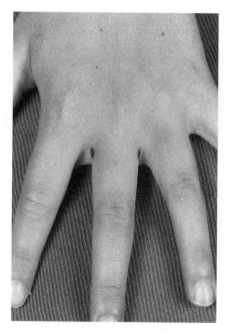

**Fig. 7.17**   Upper limb digital nerve block, injection positions.

*Indications*

For postoperative analgesia following operations on the fingers, e.g. avulsion of the nail or bony surgery to the terminal phalanx.

*Contraindication*

Local infection.

*Technique*

The nerves are easily blocked by an injection of 0.5–2 ml of local anaesthetic solution, depending on the age of the child, into the web space on each side of the digit (Figs 7.17, 7.18). The solution is then massaged around the base of the finger to produce a 'ring block' of the digital nerves. Solutions containing a vasoconstrictor **must never** be used because of the risk of gangrene of the

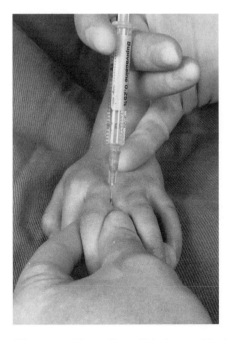

**Fig. 7.18**   Upper limb digital nerve block.

fingers. Alternatively, two injections can be made on each side in the web space, one dorsally and the other ventrally, taking care to avoid the tendons.

## REFERENCE

Moore, D. C. (1981). Digital nerve block. In *Regional block. A handbook for use in the clinical practice of medicine and surgery*, (4th edn), (ed. D. C. Moore), p. 304. Charles C. Thomas, Springfield, Illinois.

# 8

# *Intercostal nerve block*

S. J. MATHER

## Anatomy

The intercostal nerves are the ventral branches of the first 11 thoracic segmental nerves (Fig. 8.1).

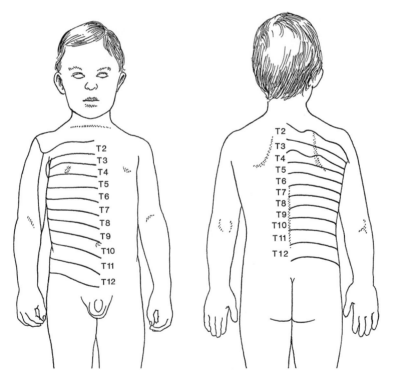

**Fig. 8.1**  Cutaneous thoracic segmental innervation.

In the paravertebral space the nerve passes very close to the pleura. At the costal angle it enters the subcostal groove. The major part of nerve runs with the blood vessels in the intercostal space, protected by the subcostal groove of the rib (Fig. 8.2). For most of their course the third, fourth, fifth and sixth nerves and vessels lie between the external and internal intercostal muscles (anteriorly) and the intercostales intimi (innermost muscle)

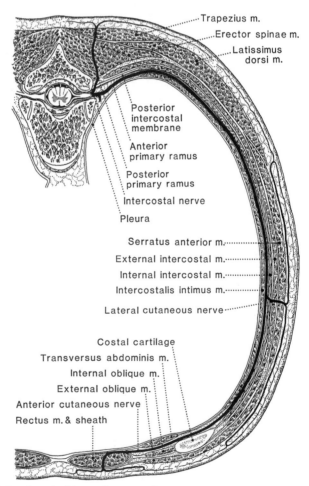

**Fig. 8.2**    A typical lower intercostal nerve.

posteriorly. The intercostales intimi separate the intercostal vessels and nerves from the pleura (these thin muscles are often absent in the upper intercostal spaces).

Close to the sternum the intercostal nerves cross in front of the internal thoracic artery, pierce the internal intercostal muscles, the external intercostal membranes, and pectoralis major. Their terminal branches form the anterior cutaneous nerves of the thorax.

The ventral rami of the tenth to eleventh thoracic nerves run anteriorly from the intercostal spaces into the abdominal wall. The terminal rami may cross the mid-line. The main branches of the intercostal nerves are:

(1) collateral branch (except first nerve);
(2) lateral cutaneous branch, which divides into anterior and posterior branches (except second nerve which becomes the intercostobrachial).

### Indications

Postoperative analgesia following thoracotomy, liver transplant or, rarely, in older children, for the pain of fractured ribs.

### Contraindications

Local infection.

### Equipment

25 g short-bevelled 2.5 cm needle and syringe of suitable size attached with extension tubing.

### Drugs

Lignocaine 0.5–1 per cent with adrenaline 1 : 200 000 or bupivacaine 0.2–0.25 per cent.

1. Absorption can be very rapid and so maximal doses should be avoided.
2. 0.5–2 ml of 0.2 or 0.25 per cent bupivacaine per segment, depending on the size of the child, is usually sufficient. Children over 50 kg should be treated as adults and 2 ml per segment of 0.375 per cent bupivacaine used.

Adrenaline-containing solutions prolong the duration of block-ade, particularly with lignocaine, but there is a risk of intravascular injection.

## *Technique*

The child lies in the lateral position with the arm alongside the head (as for thoracotomy). For rib fractures, the patient remains sitting.

The mid-line (spinous processes) is marked on the back with a skin pencil. Next, the mid-axillary line and the lower border of the rib of the segment to be blocked are marked with the pencil.

For older children, the blocks may also be performed in the posterior axillary line, which is then marked similarly.

### *Mid-axillary (lateral) approach*
The skin is marked as described above.

The needle is attached to the primed extension tube and syringe to avoid the possibility of air entering the pleural cavity from outside. It is then inserted at an angle of 80° to the chest wall, directed superiorly, toward the lower border of the upper rib of the space to be blocked.

When bone is contacted, the needle is withdrawn slightly and then slid under the rib with the bevel facing upwards (Fig. 8.3).

Loss of resistance is felt to pressure on the syringe as the space is entered.

Some anaesthetists prefer to use saline to identify the space, before local anaesthetic solution is injected. If a definite loss of resistance is not felt, the needle should not be inserted more than a further 2 mm. After careful aspiration, up to 2 ml of solution is injected in each space.

### Shelly and Park modification

Shelly and Park (1987) have described a technique which is a modification of the classical mid-axillary approach which was developed for use in children following liver transplantation. The block can be performed in either the lateral or supine position.

The mid-axillary line is used but the needle is inserted differently (Fig. 8.4).

The initial skin puncture is made perpendicular to the rib and the needle 'walked down' the rib to the inferior (caudad) edge. The needle is then re-directed posteriorly at 90° to the initial puncture line.

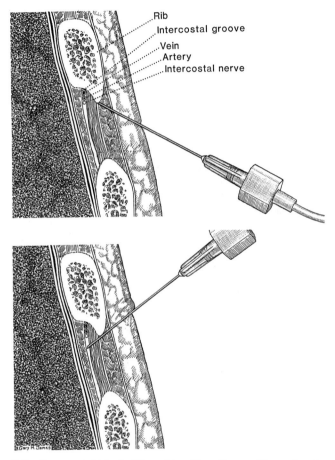

**Fig. 8.3**  Intercostal block. The mid-axillary line and lower border of the rib of the segment to be blocked are marked. A short bevelled needle (with the bevel facing upwards) and attached to a primed extension tube is inserted at 80° to the chest wall until it strikes the lower border of the upper rib of the space to be blocked. The needle is then withdrawn slightly and slid under the rib until loss of resistance is felt. (If loss of resistance is not felt after sliding the needle under the rib, the needle should be inserted no more than 2 mm). Up to 2 ml of solution is injected in each space.

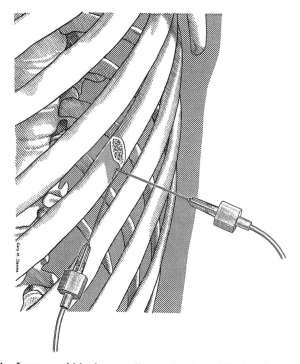

**Fig. 8.4**  Intercostal block according to Shelly and Park. The mid-axillary line is identified as before. The initial skin puncture is made *perpendicular to the rib* and the needle 'walked' down the rib to the inferior border. The needle is then angled posteriorly at 90° to the initial (perpendicular) line. The needle is advanced almost parallel to the rib, slightly medially and posteriorly until the space is identified by loss of resistance to injection.

The needle is advanced, virtually parallel to the rib, slightly medially and posteriorly until the tip lies in the subcostal groove.

The space is identified by loss of resistance as described in the classical technique above.

The advantage claimed by Shelly and Park for this technique is that the risk of pneumothorax is reduced because the needle enters the intercostal space almost parallel to the rib.

*Posterior*

A similar technique to the classic lateral approach is used.

The puncture is made at a point midway between the mid-axillary line and the spinous processes. This point equates with the posterior angle of the rib.

Intercostal blocks may also be performed by the surgeon at thoracotomy under direct vision.

## Complications

### Pneumothorax
This is more likely with the posterior approach where the nerve lies very close to the pleura.

### Intravascular injection
Careful aspiration before injection is essential.

More rarely:

### Respiratory difficulty
May be due to accidental spinal or epidural anaesthesia (dural cuffs may extend for a variable distance along the nerves).

### Local anaesthetic toxicity
This may be due to intravascular injection, intrapleural injection (where absorption can be rapid), or the injection of large doses. Because local anaesthetic agents are rapidly absorbed from this site, some anaesthetists favour the use of adrenaline-containing solutions. Submaximal doses for the size of the child should always be used. *Continuous (catheter) techniques are not recommended for children.*

Bricker *et al.* (1989) reported a series of intercostal nerve blocks in neonates and infants aged less than 6 months using 1.5 mg kg$^{-1}$ of 0.25 per cent bupivacaine (0.8 ml kg$^{-1}$). The blocks were performed under direct vision by the surgeon. Peak blood concentrations were found within 10 minutes in 18 out of 22 subjects (11 neonates and 11 infants), but no clinical adverse effects were noted. The peak whole-blood concentrations showed considerable interpatient variability, suggesting that the levels may be unpredictable and that caution should be exercised with respect to dose. Clinical experience, however, suggests that 2 mg kg$^{-1}$ is safe, even in small infants.

# REFERENCES

Bricker, S. R. W., Telford, R. J., and Booker, P. D. (1989). Pharmacokinetics of bupivacaine following intraoperative intercostal nerve block in neonates and in infants aged less than 6 months. *Anesthesiology*, **70**, 942–7.

Dalens, B. J. (1990). Intercostal nerve blocks. In *Pediatric regional anesthesia*, (ed. B. J. Dalens), p. 446. CRC Press, Boca Raton, Florida.

Shelly, M. P. and Park, G. R. (1987). Intercostal nerve blockade for children. *Anaesthesia*, **42**, 541–4.

# 9

# *Nerve blocks for inguinal herniotomy and orchidopexy*

S. J. MATHER

## ILIOINGUINAL AND ILIOHYPOGASTRIC NERVE BLOCK, GENITO-FEMORAL NERVE BLOCK

The combined ilioinguinal and iliohypogastric nerve block (iliac crest block) is one of the most useful and commonly performed blocks in paediatric anaesthesia.

### Anatomy

The ilioinguinal, iliohypogastric and genito-femoral nerves all derive from the lumbar plexus (T12, L1–L2).

The ilioinguinal nerve (T12, L1) runs below the ventral branch of the iliohypogastric nerve (T12, L1). The iliohypogastric nerve lies between the transversus abdominis and internal oblique muscles, close to the anterior superior iliac spine, and supplies the skin in the area of the inguinal ligament. The ilioinguinal nerve runs through the superficial inguinal ring to supply the skin of the scrotum in the male and the labia majora in the female.

The genito-femoral nerve (L1, L2) divides above the inguinal ligament into genital and femoral branches. The genital branch supplies the cremaster muscle and skin of the scrotum or labia majora while the femoral branch supplies the skin over the upper aspect of the front of the thigh.

### Indication

Postoperative cutaneous analgesia following hernia repair or other incision in the groin. It is important to remember that only the cutaneous innervation is blocked and therefore supplementary general anaesthesia is required unless the sac is infiltrated under direct vision by the surgeon.

For orchidopexy it is also advantageous to block the genital branch of the genito-femoral nerve in the region of the pubic tubercle. If the scrotal incision is low (in the distribution of the pudendal nerve) wound infiltration will also be necessary.

### Contraindications

Local infection; obstructed hernia.

### Equipment

Short-bevelled 23 or 25 g 2.5 cm needle and syringe.

### Drugs

Up to 2.5 mg kg$^{-1}$ of bupivacaine 0.25 or 0.5 per cent. For bilateral blocks the 0.5 per cent solution should be diluted so as not to exceed 2.5 mg kg$^{-1}$. 0.25 per cent provides satisfactory analgesia in the younger child.

In teenagers 0.5 per cent may be used (diluted for bilateral blocks). The stronger solution is more likely to produce unwanted motor block of the femoral nerve, which has been reported.

### Duration of action

This is shorter than is generally appreciated (2–3 hours). Supplementary oral or rectal analgesia should be prescribed to be given regularly for 24 hours.

### Technique 1

The child's index finger is used to gauge the distance medial from the iliac spine where the puncture is made.

One (child's) finger breadth above and medial to the anterior superior iliac spine (point X1 in Fig. 9.1) a *short-bevelled* needle, *without the syringe attached,* is placed at right angles to the skin until a 'pop' is felt as the needle pierces the external oblique aponeurosis.

The needle, when released, should stand up unsupported. If it falls to one side or other, the needle point is outside the aponeurosis.

When the needle is in the correct position the syringe is attached and one-third of the volume deposited beneath the aponeurosis. The needle is then withdrawn until the tip is subcutaneous as a further third of the solution is injected, so as to infiltrate the muscle layer and the subcutaneous tissue in a 90° 'fan' medial from the iliac crest.

The remainder of the solution is then injected subcutaneously in the mid-line from the symphysis pubis to a point which is one-third of the distance from the symphysis to the umbilicus.

If an orchidopexy is being performed, 1–2 ml of the total volume should be reserved for infiltration adjacent to the pubic tubercle just above the inguinal ligament (point X2 in Fig. 9.1) in an attempt to block the genital branch of the genito-femoral nerve.

Most surgeons find no difficulty in carrying out herniotomy when the block is done preoperatively, but it may also be performed at the end of the procedure. This may be disadvantageous in that the block may take up to 20 minutes to be fully effective.

### Technique 2

In this technique, described by several authors, the needle is directed in different directions in an attempt to block each nerve in turn.

The needle is inserted a (child's) finger's breadth medial to the anterior superior iliac spine and directed posterolaterally until it strikes bone.

The needle is then withdrawn very slightly (so as not to make a subperiosteal injection) and an injection of 0.25 or 0.5 per cent bupivacaine ($0.5–1$ mg kg$^{-1}$) made as the needle is withdrawn to the subcutaneous tissue.

Since the iliohypogastric and ilioinguinal nerves run close together, the ilioinguinal nerve may be partially (but not reliably) blocked.

A further injection of $0.5–1$ mg kg$^{-1}$ is then made with the needle directed toward the inguinal ring, the short-bevelled needle having been inserted through the external oblique aponeurosis. The solution should be injected both above and below the muscle, as the needle is withdrawn.

The remainder of the solution (total dose 2.5 mg kg$^{-1}$) should then be infiltrated in the mid-line or used to block the genital branch of the genito-femoral nerve, as in Technique 1.

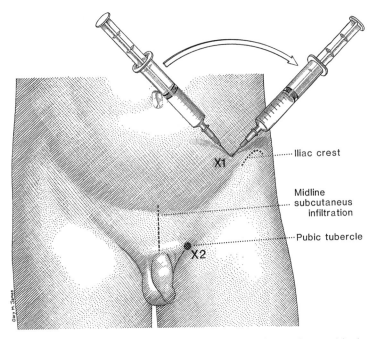

**Fig. 9.1** Ilioinguinal, iliohypogastric, and genito-femoral nerve blocks (technique 2). To block the ilioinguinal and iliohypogastric nerves the needle is inserted one (child's) finger breadth medial to the anterior superior iliac spine (X1) and directed posterolaterally until it strikes bone. It is then withdrawn slightly and the injection made as the needle is withdrawn to a subcutaenous position. The needle is then reinserted through the external oblique aponeurosis (a slight 'click' should be felt) and further solution injected both above and below the aponeurosis as the needle is withdrawn. For orchidopexy, one-third of the total volume should be injected in each manoeuvre, with the remaining third deposited adjacent to the pubic tubercle, above the inguinal ligament (X2). Because nerve fibres may cross the mid-line, it is desirable to infiltrate the subcutaneous tissues for a few centimetres upwards from the symphysis pubis.

## REFERENCES

Roy-Shapira, A., Amoury, R. A., Ashcraft, K. W., Holder, T. M., and Sharp, R. J. (1985). Transient quadriceps paresis following local inguinal block for post-operative pain control. *Journal of Paediatric Surgery*, **20**, 554–5.

Shandling, B. and Stewart, D. J. (1980). Regional analgesia for post-operative pain in paediatric out-patient surgery. *Journal Paediatric Surgery*, **15**, 477.

Yaster, M. and Maxwell, L. G. (1989). Pediatric regional anesthesia. *Anesthesiology*, **70**, 324–38.

# 10

## *Penile block*

J. M. PEUTRELL

### Anatomy

*The nerve supply to the penis*

The penis is supplied by sensory nerves from the lumbo-sacral plexus and autonomic fibres from the inferior hypogastric plexus:

(1) the two dorsal nerves of the penis innervate the glans and the distal two-thirds of the body of the penis;

(2) the ilioinguinal and genito-femoral nerves supply the base of the penis;

(3) autonomic fibres accompany either the dorsal nerves or the blood vessels.

The dorsal nerves of the penis (S2–S4) arise as terminal branches of the pudendal nerves. They run along the ischial ramus and then the lower border of the pubic ramus. They enter the subpubic space (see below) by passing between the perineal membrane and the inferior pubic ligament. Within the subpubic space the dorsal nerves run on the corpus cavernosum and pass into the root of the penis deep to the penile fascia (Buck's fascia). Within the penis the dorsal nerves lie at the 10 and 2 o'clock positions lateral to the two dorsal penile arteries and the mid-line dorsal veins (superficial and deep) (Fig. 10.1). The nerves divide into smaller subcutaneous branches just beyond the root of the penis to supply the dorsum of the penis. Ventral branches supplying the ventral penis and frenulum arise from the dorsal nerves early in the course within the subpubic space.

The dorsal penile nerves can be blocked at three sites: within the subpubic space, beneath the penile fascia at the root of the penis, or as the terminal divisions run subcutaneously.

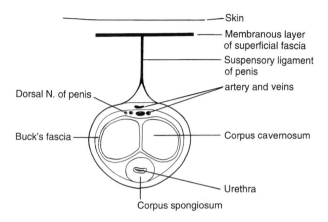

**Fig. 10.1**   Cross-section of the root of the penis, showing the nerves lying lateral to the arteries deep to the penile fascia and the superficial and deep veins lying in the mid-line.

The ventral penile nerves may be included in blocks within the subpubic space. They are also blocked by a subcutaneous injection at the junction between the ventral surface of the penis and the scrotum.

*The subpubic space*

As the nerves emerge from beneath the pubic ramus they are enclosed within a fat-filled space termed the 'subpubic space'. The boundaries of the subpubic space are (Fig. 10.2):

(1)  postero-superiorly—the pubic bone and perineal membrane;
(2)  postero-inferiorly—the horizontal part of the corpus cavernosa and its enclosing fascia (continuous with the penile fascia at the root of the penis); and
(3)  anteriorly—deep layer of the superficial fascia of the anterior abdominal wall (Scarpa's fascia) which is continuous with the penile fascia, the superficial layer of the superficial fascia and the skin over the pubic area.

The subpubic space is separated by the suspensory ligament of the penis into left and right compartments.

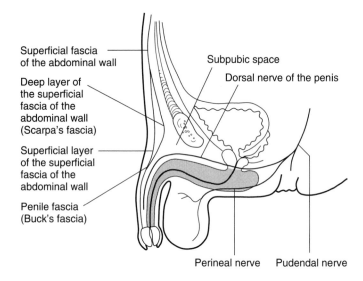

**Fig. 10.2** The course of the branches of the pudendal nerve and the relations of the subpubic space. (Based on and adapted from figure 1 from Dalens, B. *et al.* (1989). Penile block via the subpubic space in 100 children. *Anesthesia Analgesia*, **69**, 41–5).

### Indications

(1) circumcision;

(2) distal hypospadias repair—block of the dorsal nerves of the penis is not effective for proximal hypospadias repair. The proximal ventral penis and adjacent perineum are innervated by the ilioinguinal, genito-femoral, and the ventral branches of the dorsal nerves of the penis.

METHODS OF PENILE BLOCK

Techniques blocking the dorsal nerves within the penile fascia at the root of the penis have the potential to cause bleeding, usually from the dorsal veins. A haematoma confined within the penile fascia may compress the arterial supply to the penis and cause gangrene. Subcutaneous ring block of the penis and block of the penile nerve within the subpubic space (Fig. 10.3) are simple techniques unlikely to damage important structures or cause a significant haematoma.

## Subcutaneous ring block of the penis

The advantages of the subcutaneous ring block of the penis are:

(1) the technique is simple and needs no special training;
(2) any bleeding will not cause a haematoma within a confined space;
(3) the technique avoids the dorsal blood vessels and the corpus cavernosum.

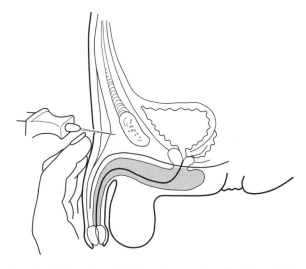

**Fig. 10.3** A sagittal view through the perineum showing the technique of penile block within the subpubic space (based on figure 4B from Dalens, B. *et al.* (1989). Penile block via the subpubic space in 100 children. *Anesthesia Analgesia*, **69**, 41–5).

The efficacy of the subcutaneous ring block has not been compared with the techniques that block the penile nerve within the subpubic space (see below) or at the root of the penis.

## Equipment

2.5 cm 25 g needle for subcutaneous injection.

## Drugs

Bupivacaine 0.25 per cent sufficient to produce an obvious skin weal (1.5–5.0 ml in total, depending on the size of the child). Adrenaline should NEVER be injected into the penis.

## Complications

Superficial haematoma.

## Technique

The boy lies supine. The skin at the root of the penis is cleaned with an alcoholic antiseptic solution. The penis is held between the thumb and forefinger of the non-dominant hand. Local anaesthetic is infiltrated subcutaneously in a ring at the base of the penis in a volume sufficient to produce an obvious weal (Fig. 10.4).

A larger volume of local anaesthetic is injected in the mid-line dorsally than elsewhere (Fig. 10.5). Care is taken to avoid obvious blood vessels.

## Penile block within the subpubic space

The advantages of block of the dorsal penile nerves within the subpubic space are:

(1) vascular structures (e.g. corpus cavernosum, dorsal arteries and veins) are less likely to be damaged;
(2) nerve damage is unlikely because local anaesthetic is delivered into a space rather than immediately adjacent to the nerve;
(3) the subpubic space is relatively large and the volume of local anaesthetic or a haematoma is unlikely to compress the penile arteries.

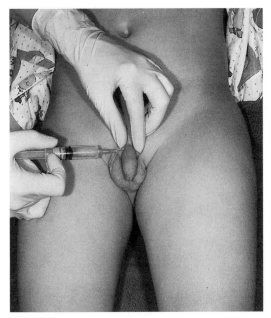

**Fig. 10.4** Subcutaneous ring block of the penis. Local anaesthetic is infiltrated subcutaneously in a ring at the base of the penis in a volume sufficient to produce an obvious weal.

### Equipment
2.5 or 5.0 cm short-bevelled needles (depending upon the thickness of subcutaneous fat).

### Drugs
Bupivacaine 0.5 per cent 0.1 ml kg$^{-1}$ for each subpubic injection (total of 0.2 ml kg$^{-1}$ = 1 mg kg$^{-1}$). Adrenaline should NEVER be used for blocks of the penis.

### Duration of action
5 hours or longer.

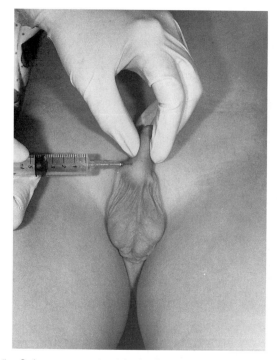

**Fig. 10.5**   Subcutaneous ring block of the penis. A larger volume of local anaesthetic is injected in the mid-line dorsally than elsewhere. Care is taken to avoid obvious blood vessels.

## Complications

The main complication is advancing the needle too far and puncturing the corpus cavernosum or dorsal vessels. Compression of the arteries and ischaemia of the penis is unlikely unless the haematoma is very large. Intravascular injection of local anaesthetic may produce systemic toxicity.

## Techniques

The boy lies supine. The skin over the pubic bone is cleaned with an alcoholic antiseptic solution. The point of needle insertion is 0.5 cm (babies) and 1.0 cm (older boys) lateral to the symphysis

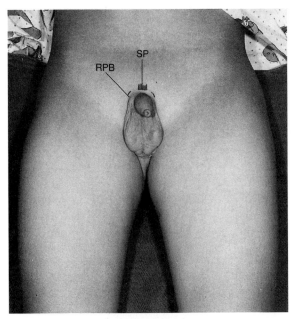

**Fig. 10.6**　Penile block within the subpubic space. The point of needle insertion is 0.5 cm (babies) and 1.0 cm (older boys) lateral to the symphysis pubis (SP) immediately below the right (RPB) and left inferior rami of the pubic bone.

pubis (SP) immediately below the right (RPB) and left inferior rami of the pubic bone (Fig. 10.6).

The penis is held between the thumb and forefinger of the non-dominant hand and the base of the penis is pulled gently down. The needle is inserted and advanced posteriorly, slightly caudally (10–20° to the transverse plane) and slightly medially (10–20° to the sagittal plane) (Fig. 10.7).

A 'pop' is felt twice as the needle tip penetrates first the superficial layer of the superficial fascia and then Scarpa's fascia. The subpubic space lies deep to Scarpa's fascia, 8–30 mm from the skin. The depth of the space does not correlate with age or weight. After aspiration local anaesthetic is injected slowly (Fig. 10.8).

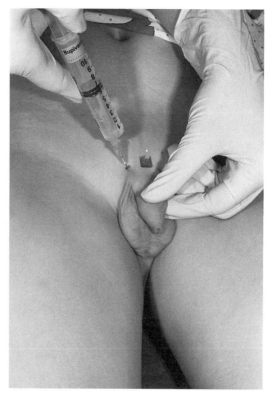

**Fig. 10.7**  Penile block within the subpubic space. The needle is inserted and advanced posteriorly, slightly caudally (10–20° to the transverse plane) and slightly medially (10–20° to the sagittal plane).

The rate of success of the subpubic block is increased by also blocking the ventral nerves of the penis. Local anaesthetic is injected subcutaneously at the junction between the ventral penis and the scrotum (see Fig. 10.5) in a volume that produces an obvious skin weal.

## REFERENCES

Blaise, G. and Roy, W. L. (1986). Postoperative pain relief after hypospadias repair in pediatric patients: regional analgesia versus systemic analgesics. *Anesthesiology*, **65**, 84–6.

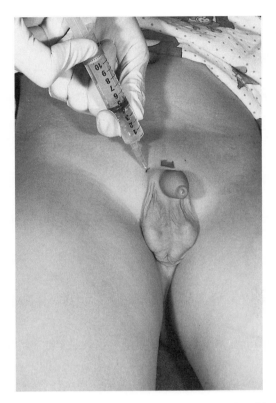

**Fig. 10.8**  Penile block within the subpubic space. A 'pop' is felt twice as the needle tip penetrates first the superficial layer of the superficial fascia and then Scarpa's fascia. The subpubic space lies deep to Scarpa's fascia, 8–30 mm from the skin. After aspiration local anaesthetic is injected slowly.

Broadman, L. M., Hannallah, R. S., Belman, A. B., Elder, P. T., Ruttimann, U., and Epstein, B. S. (1987). Post-circumcision analgesia—a prospective evaluation of subcutaneous ring block of the penis. *Anesthesiology*, **67**, 399–402.

Brown, T. C. K., Weidner, N. J., and Bouwmeester, J. (1989). Dorsal nerve of penis block—anatomical and radiological studies. *Anaesthesia Intensive Care*, **17**, 34–8.

Dalens, B., Vanneuville, G., and Dechelotte, P. (1989). Penile block via the subpubic space in 100 children. *Anesthesia Analgesia*, **69**, 41–5.

Sara, C. A. and Lowry, C. J. (1984). A complication of circumcision and dorsal block of the penis. *Anaesthesia Intensive Care*, **13**, 79–85.

Serour, F., Mori, J., and Barr, J. (1994). Optimal regional anesthesia for circumcision. *Anesthesia Analgesia*, **79**, 129–31.

# 11

# *Nerve blocks of the lower limb*

## J. M. PEUTRELL

## SCIATIC NERVE

*Anatomy*

The sciatic nerve (L4–S3) leaves the pelvis through the greater sciatic foramen accompanied by the posterior cutaneous nerve of the thigh and then passes beneath piriformis. In the buttock it lies half-way between the greater trochanter and the ischial tuberosity covered by gluteus maximus. The sciatic nerve enters the back of the thigh by passing deep to the long head of biceps femoris and descends towards the apex of the popliteal fossa. It divides into its terminal divisions (tibial and common peroneal nerves) in the lower third of the thigh.

The sciatic nerve innervates the hip and its peroneal and tibial divisions supply sensation to (Fig. 11.1a, b):

(1) the skin of most of the lower leg and the foot;
(2) the knee, ankle, and foot joints.

The posterior cutaneous nerve of the thigh accompanies the sciatic nerve in the buttock but passes superficial to biceps femoris. It supplies the skin of the posterior thigh and the back of the knee. It may be included in blocks of the sciatic nerve in the hip or buttock but not in the thigh.

*Indications*

Operations on the lower leg, foot, or knee (usually combined with other nerve blocks, e.g. femoral, lateral cutaneous, or saphenous nerves).

142

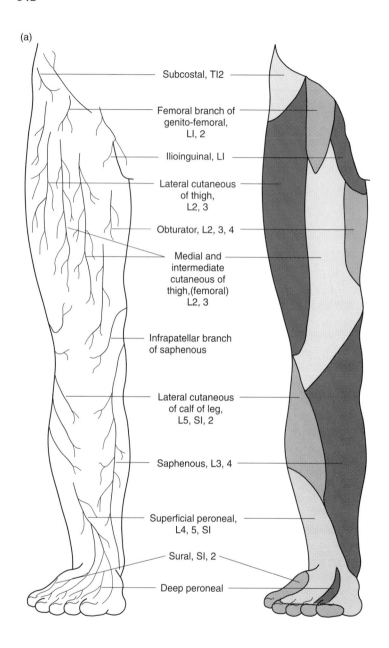

**Fig. 11.1** Cutaneous innervation of (a) anterior leg and (b) posterior leg.

(b)

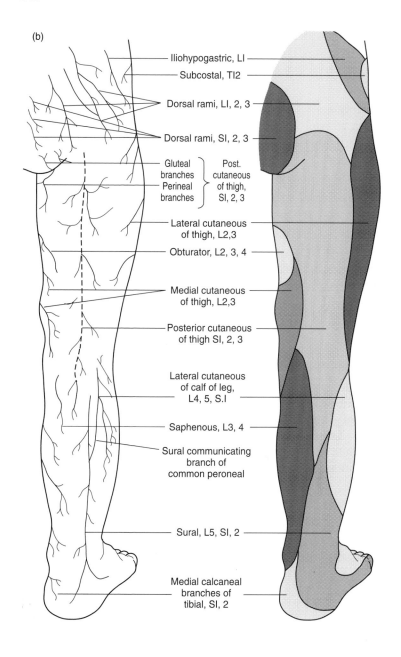

Iliohypogastric, LI
Subcostal, TI2
Dorsal rami, LI, 2, 3
Dorsal rami, SI, 2, 3

Gluteal branches
Perineal branches
Post. cutaneous of thigh, SI, 2, 3

Lateral cutaneous of thigh, L2,3
Obturator, L2, 3, 4
Medial cutaneous of thigh, L2,3
Posterior cutaneous of thigh SI, 2, 3
Lateral cutaneous of calf of leg, L4, 5, S.I
Saphenous, L3, 4
Sural communicating branch of common peroneal
Sural, L5, SI, 2
Medial calcaneal branches of tibial, SI, 2

## Contraindications

Local infection, coagulopathy.

## Drugs

Bupivacaine 0.5 per cent 2.0 mg kg$^{-1}$ (0.4 ml kg$^{-1}$). The concentration of bupivacaine should be reduced to decrease the risk of toxicity if other major nerves are also blocked.

## Duration of action

The duration of analgesia after a successful nerve block is at least 4 hours, and in many children is greater than 12 hours.

## Complications

Rarely dysaesthesia, hypoaesthesia, or motor weakness (foot drop).

## METHODS OF SCIATIC NERVE BLOCK

### Posterior approach in the buttock (Raj *et al.* 1975)

There are well-defined landmarks and this method is technically straightforward. The posterior cutaneous nerve of the thigh is sometimes blocked along with the sciatic nerve in the buttock (see below). The disadvantage of this technique is that the leg must be positioned properly and therefore it is not suitable if the leg has severe injuries.

## Equipment

(1)  22 g 50 mm needle suitable for use with a nerve stimulator;
(2)  tubing to connect between the needle and syringe;
(3)  a peripheral nerve stimulator.

## Technique

The needle is inserted half-way between the greater trochanter of the femur and the ischial tuberosity (Figs 11.2, 11.3).

The child lies supine with the leg held flexed at the hip. The skin is cleaned with an alcoholic antiseptic solution. The needle is inserted at right angles to the skin and advanced slowly until stim-

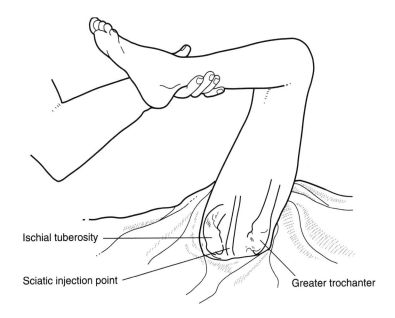

**Fig. 11.2**   Landmarks for sciatic nerve block in the buttock.

ulation with the peripheral nerve stimulator produces plantar or dorsiflexion of the foot.

**Anterior approach at the hip**

This technique is more complicated but has the advantage that the leg does not need to be moved. Block of the posterior cutaneous nerve of the thigh is sometimes included. The failure rate is about 5 per cent.

*Equipment*

(1)  22 g 50–80 mm needle with a short bevel (e.g. a lumbar puncture or insulated local block needle);

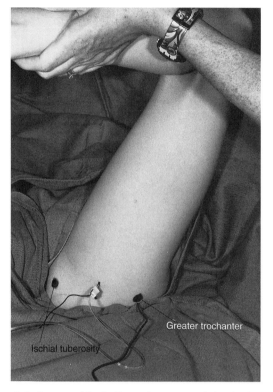

**Fig. 11.3**   Sciatic nerve block. Posterior approach in the buttock
(Raj 1975).

(2)   ('nerve stimulation technique') peripheral nerve stimulator;
(3)   ('loss of resistance technique') 10 ml syringe containing
      0.9 per cent sodium chloride.

*Technique*

The child lies supine. The skin is cleaned with an alcoholic antiseptic antiseptic solution. The landmarks for the anterior approach to the sciatic nerve are shown (Fig. 11.4). The line drawn
from the anterior superior iliac spine to the pubic tubercle indicates the position of the inguinal ligament (Fig. 11.5).

This line is trisected and a perpendicular dropped from the
junction of the medial one-third and lateral two-thirds. A second

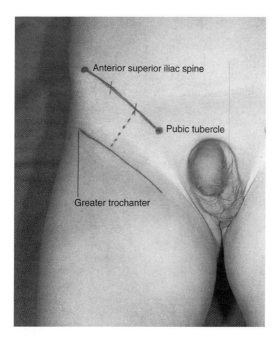

**Fig. 11.4**   Landmarks for block of the sciatic nerve at the hip using an anterior approach.

line is drawn from the greater trochanter parallel to the inguinal ligament.

The needle is inserted at the point where the perpendicular meets the line from the greater trochanter (Fig. 11.6). It is advanced at right angles to the skin in a sagittal plane and slightly laterally. The position of the nerve can be identified either by 'loss of resistance' or with a peripheral nerve stimulator:

*Anterior approach in children using a loss of resistance technique (McNicol 1985)*

When the needle tip hits the femur it is redirected and 'walked off' the medial edge of the femur. A 10 ml syringe containing 0.9 per cent sodium chloride is attached to the needle. Light pressure is applied through the barrel of the syringe as the needle is advanced deeper through muscle. There is loss of resistance to injection as the needle tip enters the compartment containing the

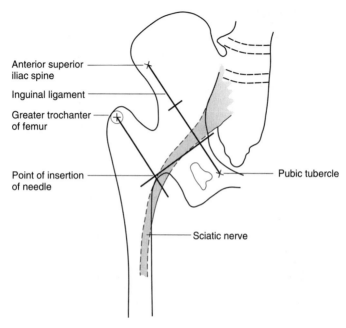

**Fig. 11.5**   Sciatic nerve block, anterior approach at the hip.

sciatic nerve. After aspirating for blood, local anaesthetic is injected and the needle removed.

*Anterior approach using a nerve stimulator*
The needle is 'walked off' the medial edge of the femur and the sciatic nerve located with a peripheral nerve stimulator. Local anaesthetic is injected when a current from the peripheral nerve stimulator of 0.5 mA or less causes dorsiflexion or plantar flexion of the foot.

## Posterior approach in the thigh

This technique (attributed to McKenzie by Brown and Fisk 1992) is straightforward but has the disadvantages that it does not block the articular branches to the hip or the posterior cutaneous nerve of the thigh, and the leg must be moved.

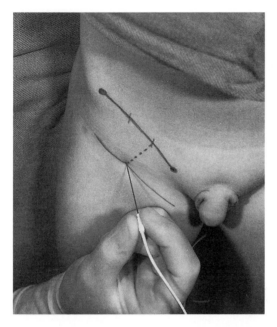

**Fig. 11.6** Sciatic nerve block, anterior approach at the hip. The needle is inserted at the point where the perpendicular meets the line from the greater trochanter. It is advanced at right angles to the skin in a sagittal plane and slightly laterally. The position of the nerve can be identified either by 'loss of resistance' or with a peripheral nerve stimulator.

*Equipment*

(1)   22 g 50 mm needle suitable for use with a nerve stimulator;
(2)   tubing to connect between the needle and syringe;
(3)   a peripheral nerve stimulator.

*Technique*

The child lies supine with the leg flexed at the hip. The skin is cleaned with an alcoholic antiseptic solution. The position of needle insertion is at the mid-point of a line drawn from the ischial tuberosity to the head of the fibula (Figs 11.7, 11.8).

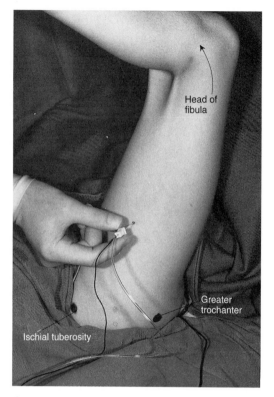

**Fig. 11.7** Sciatic nerve block, posterior approach in the thigh.

The needle is advanced at right angles to the skin. The depth of the sciatic nerve is indicated by loss of resistance as the needle tip emerges deep to biceps femoris. Local anaesthetic is injected when dorsiflexion or plantar flexion of the foot is produced by a current from the peripheral nerve stimulator of 0.5 mA or less.

## REFERENCES

Brown, T. C. K., and Fisk, G. C. (1992). Regional and local anaesthesia. In *Anaesthesia for children*, (2nd edn), pp. 315–16. Blackwell Scientific Publications, Oxford.

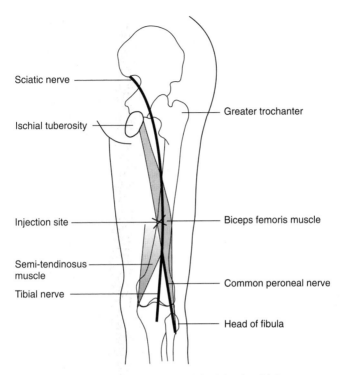

**Fig. 11.8**   Landmarks for sciatic nerve block in the thigh.

McNicol, L. R. (1985). Sciatic nerve block for children. *Anaesthesia*, **40**, 410–14.

Raj, P. P., Parks, R. I., Watson, T. D., and Jenkins, M. T. (1975). New single-position supine approach to sciatic-femoral nerve block. *Anesthesia Analgesia*, **54**, 489–93.

# POSTERIOR CUTANEOUS NERVE OF THE THIGH

*Anatomy*

The posterior femoral cutaneous nerve of the thigh (S1–S3) leaves the pelvis through the greater sciatic foramen posterior or

medial to the sciatic nerve. It is generally closely associated with
the sciatic nerve in the buttock but can separate quite early in its
curve. It lies deep to piriformis and is covered by gluteus maximus
in the buttock but passes superficial to the long head of biceps
femoris. It supplies cutaneous branches to the perineum, lower
lateral buttock, back of the thigh, popliteal fossa and the upper
part of the back of the lower leg (Fig. 11.1).

### Indications

Operations on the back of the thigh or the popliteal fossa.

### Technique

The nerve is usually closely associated with the sciatic nerve in
the buttock and can be included in blocks of the sciatic nerve at
the hip or buttock. It is separated from the sciatic nerve in the
thigh by the long head of biceps femoris and is not included in the
technique attributed to McKenzie (see above).


## FEMORAL NERVE

### Anatomy

The femoral nerve (L2–L4) arises from the lumbar plexus. It
emerges at the lateral border of psoas to descend in the groove
between the psoas and iliacus muscles lying deep to the fascia iliaca.
The nerve enters the groin by passing beneath the inguinal ligament lateral to the femoral artery (Fig. 11.9) from which it is
separated by a fibrous septum from the fascia iliaca (Fig. 11.10).

The femoral nerve contains motor and sensory fibres. It innervates the quadriceps muscle and supplies sensation to the skin of
the anterior thigh, medial part of the knee, medial aspect of the
calf (Fig. 11.1) and the periosteum of the femur.

### Indications

(1) Operations on the hip or femur (combined with block of the
    lateral femoral cutaneous nerve of the thigh);
(2) superficial operations of anterior thigh or medial calf (e.g.
    skin grafting and muscle biopsy);

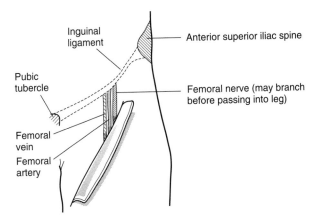

**Fig. 11.9**   Anatomy of the femoral nerve.

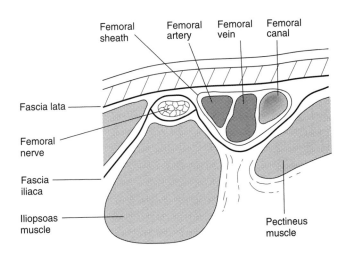

**Fig. 11.10**   Cross-section of the groin showing the relationship of the femoral nerve to the femoral vessels and the fascia iliaca and fascia lata.

(3) operations on the knee (combined with blocks of the sciatic and lateral cutaneous nerves of the thigh);

(4) fractured shaft of femur—pain relief is obtained because the block produces analgesia of the periosteum and stops spasm of the quadriceps muscle.

## Contraindications

Local sepsis, coagulopathy.

## Equipment

5.0 cm 22 or 24 g short-bevelled needles, peripheral nerve stimulator.

## Drugs

Bupivacaine 0.5 per cent 0.2–0.4 ml kg$^{-1}$ ( = 1.0–2.0 mg kg$^{-1}$). The concentration of bupivacaine should be reduced if other major nerves are also blocked.

## Onset of block

Within 10 minutes.

## Duration of action

About 6 hours.

## Complications

Haematoma; intravascular injection producing systemic toxicity; (rarely) damage of the femoral nerve producing dysaesthesia, hypoaesthesia, and weakness of the quadriceps muscle.

## Technique

The child lies supine. The skin is cleaned with an alcoholic antiseptic solution. A line drawn between the anterior superior iliac spine and pubic tubercle indicates the position of the inguinal ligament (Fig. 11.11). The needle is inserted 0.5–1.0 cm below the inguinal ligament, 0.5–1.0 cm lateral to the pulsations of the femoral artery (Fig. 11.12).

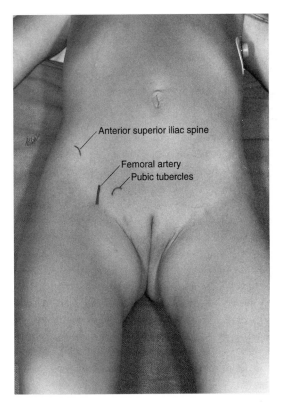

**Fig. 11.11**    Femoral nerve block. A line drawn between the anterior superior iliac spine and pubic tubercle indicates the position of the inguinal ligament.

The needle is advanced 40° to the skin in a sagittal plane aiming in a rostral direction until the peripheral nerve stimulator produces contractions of the quadriceps muscle. The needle is repositioned until contractions are produced with a current of 0.5 mA or less. The needle is aspirated and local anaesthetic then injected slowly.

If a peripheral nerve stimulator is not used, the plane in which the nerve lies can be found by feeling a 'pop' or loss of resistance twice as the needle penetrates the fascia lata and fascia iliaca. Local anaesthetic is injected immediately deep to the fascia iliaca.

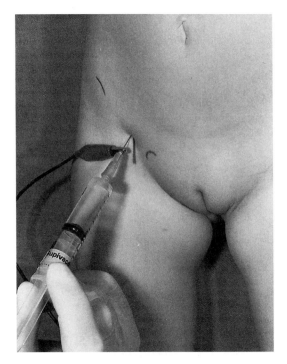

**Fig. 11.12**    Femoral nerve block. The needle is inserted 0.5–1.0 cm
below the inguinal ligament, 0.5–1.0 cm lateral to the pulsations of the
femoral artery.

## REFERENCES

Dalens, B., Vanneuville, G., and Tanguy, A. (1989). Comparison of the
    fascia iliaca compartment block with the 3-in-1 block in children.
    *Anesthesia Analgesia*, **69**, 705–13.
McNicol, L. R. (1986). Lower limb blocks for children. *Anaesthesia*, **41**,
    27–31.
Rhonchi, L. *et al.* (1989). Femoral nerve blockade in children using
    bupivacaine. *Anesthesiology*, **70**, 622–4.

## LATERAL CUTANEOUS NERVE OF THE THIGH

### Anatomy

The lateral cutaneous nerve of the thigh (L2–L3) arises from the
lumbar plexus. It emerges from the lateral border of psoas to run

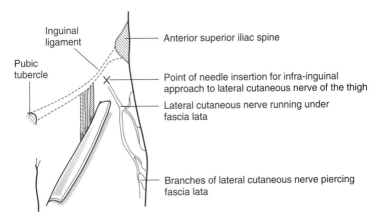

**Fig. 11.13**    Anatomy of the lateral cutaneous nerve of the thigh.

obliquely towards the anterior superior iliac spine lying between iliacus muscle and fascia iliaca. The nerve passes behind or through the inguinal ligament about a finger breadth medial to the anterior spine (Fig. 11.13) and enters the thigh lying deep to the fascia lata. It divides into anterior and posterior branches. The anterior branch perforates the fascia lata to supply the skin of the anterolateral thigh as far as the knee and contributes branches to the patellar plexus. The posterior branch perforates the fascia lata at a higher level and passes backwards to supply the skin of the lateral thigh between the greater trochanter and the middle of the thigh (Fig. 11.14).

The lateral cutaneous nerve of the thigh has no motor fibres and cannot be identified with a peripheral nerve stimulator.

## Indications

The lateral cutaneous nerve of the thigh is often blocked in conjunction with the femoral nerve to provide analgesia for:

(1)  lateral incisions of the thigh for operations on the hip or femur (with incisions below the level of the greater trochanter);
(2)  superficial operations of lateral thigh (including skin grafting);
(3)  operations on the knee.

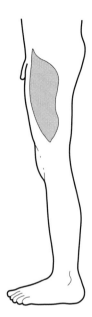

**Fig. 11.14** Lateral thigh showing the area of skin supplied by the lateral cutaneous nerve of the thigh.

*Equipment*

2.5 cm 24 g short-bevelled needle.

*Drugs*

Bupivacaine 0.5 per cent 0.1–0.2 ml kg$^{-1}$ (= 0.5–1.0 mg kg$^{-1}$). The concentration should be reduced to decrease the risk of toxicity if other major nerves are also blocked.

*Duration of action*

Four hours or longer.

*Complications*

Rarely, dysaesthesia or hypoaesthesia.

## Infra-inguinal approach

### *Technique*

The child lies supine. The skin is cleaned with an alcoholic antiseptic solution. A line drawn from the anterior superior iliac spine to the pubic tubercle indicates the position of the inguinal ligament. The needle is inserted about 1.0 cm medial to the anterior superior iliac spine and below the inguinal ligament (Fig. 11.15). The needle is advanced in the sagittal plane at an angle of 60° to the skin, aiming rostrally. A 'pop' is felt as the needle penetrates the fascia lata. Local anaesthetic is injected immediately deep to the fascia lata.

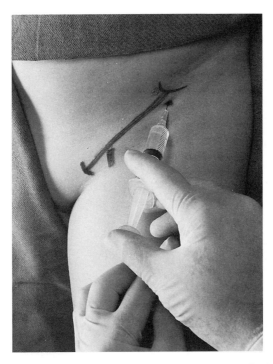

**Fig. 11.15**    Lateral cutaneous nerve of the thigh. The infra-inguinal approach to nerve block.

## Supra-inguinal approach

*Technique*

The child lies supine. The skin is cleaned with an alcoholic anti-septic solution. The needle is inserted immediately medial to the anterior superior iliac spine above the inguinal ligament (Fig. 11.16). The needle is advanced slightly medially and cau-dally. A loss of resistance is felt twice as the aponeurosis of the external oblique and the insertion of the internal oblique muscles are penetrated. Local anaesthetic is injected immediately deep to the internal oblique.

## REFERENCES

McNicol, L. R. (1986). Lower limb blocks for children. *Anaesthesia*, **41**, 27–31.

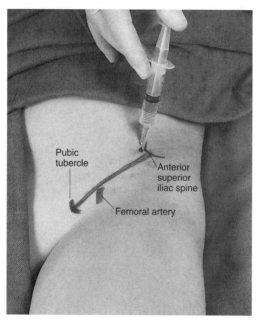

**Fig. 11.16**  Lateral cutaneous nerve of the thigh. The supra-inguinal approach to nerve block.

## OBTURATOR NERVE

*Anatomy*

The obturator nerve (L2–L4) arises from the lumbar plexus and descends through psoas to emerge from its medial border at the pelvic brim. It descends on the lateral wall of the lesser pelvis accompanied by the common and internal iliac vessels. The obturator nerve enters the thigh through the upper part of the obturator foramen where it divides into anterior and posterior branches. The anterior division gives an articular branch to the hip joint and innervates the skin of the medial thigh. The posterior division supplies an articular branch to the knee joint. Both divisions innervate the adductor muscles of the hip.

*Indications*

Operations on the hip or knee joints.

*Technique*

Finding the obturator nerve within the obturator foramen is difficult but the nerve is blocked as part of the 'fascia iliaca compartment block' described by Dalens and colleagues (see below).

## THE FASCIA ILIACA BLOCK

The 'fascia iliaca compartment block' was developed by Dalens and colleagues from post-mortem and radiological studies in children. The femoral, obturator, and lateral cutaneous nerves of the thigh are blocked with a single injection of local anaesthetic.

The technique has several advantages over other methods.

(1) nerve damage is unlikely because nerves are not sought with a needle;

(2) the rate of successful block of all three nerves in children (femoral, obturator, and lateral cutaneous nerves of the thigh) is much higher compared with the 'three in one' paravascular technique described by Winnie and colleagues (Winnie *et al.* 1973);

(3)  A catheter can be threaded into the fascia iliaca compartment
      and used to give increments of local anaesthetic to extend
      the duration of analgesia.

## Anatomy

The fascia iliaca is a complex but delicate fascia overlying the
psoas and iliacus muscles and forming the roof of a potential
space known as the 'fascia iliaca compartment'. The compartment
is limited medially by the fusion of the fascia iliaca with the psoas
sheath. The femoral, obturator, genito-femoral and lateral
cutaneous nerves of the thigh pass from the lumbar plexus to run
for a significant distance within the fascia iliaca compartment
lying deep to the fascia iliaca. The fascia iliaca is tightly attached
to the iliac crest and pelvic brim and at the groin is continuous
with the deeper layers of the inguinal ligament and the psoas
sheath. In the thigh it is tough and lies deep to the fascia lata
separating iliopsoas from sartorius laterally, and the femoral
sheath (containing the femoral artery and vein) medially. Inferior
to the inguinal ligament the fascia iliaca forms the roof of a fat-
filled space known as the 'lacuna musculorum'. The lacuna
musculorum is continuous superiorly with the fascia iliaca compartment. Local anaesthetic injected into the lacuna musculorum
should spread to block all the nerves passing through the fascia
iliaca compartment.

## Indications

(1)  Operations on the hip with incisions below the level of the
      greater trochanter;
(2)  operations on the knee (combined with a sciatic nerve
      block);
(3)  fracture of the femur;
(4)  superficial operations on the anterior and lateral thigh (e.g.
      skin grafting).

## Equipment

*Single injection of local anaesthetic*
2.5 cm 24 g short-bevelled needle with extension tubing.

*Catheter technique*

A cannula with a short-bevelled or bullet-shaped tip and a catheter that will thread through the cannula (e.g. the Contiplex® catheter set manufactured by B. Braun Med Ltd or the brachial plexus set manufactured by Arrow® International, Inc).

*Drugs*

Lignocaine with 1 in 200 000 adrenaline and bupivacaine can be used alone or in combination. Local anaesthetic is injected in a volume according to weight (Table 11.1). The concentration should be reduced if the sciatic nerve is also blocked.

**Table 11.1**  Fascia iliaca compartment block: total volume of a local anaesthetic using either: 1% lignocaine with adrenaline 1 : 200 000 or 0.5% lignocaine and 0.25% bupivacaine with 1 : 200 000 adrenaline or 0.25% bupivacaine (Dalens *et al.* 1989).

| Weight of child (kg) | Total volume of local anaesthetic |
|---|---|
| < 20 | 0.7 ml kg$^{-1}$ |
| 20–30 | 15 ml |
| 30–40 | 20 ml |
| 40–50 | 25 ml |
| > 50 | 27.5 ml |

*Duration of action*

The duration of block using a solution of 0.5 per cent lignocaine and 0.25 per cent bupivacaine with 1 in 200 000 adrenaline is about 5 hours. The duration of analgesia is slightly shorter compared with the technique of 'three in one' block described by Winnie *et al.* (Dalens *et al.* 1989). This is probably explained by a greater spread of local anaesthetic in a more vascular area.

*Complications*

There are no reported complications.

*Technique*

The child lies supine. The skin is cleaned with an alcoholic anti-septic solution. The position of the inguinal ligament is indicated by a line drawn between the anterior superior iliac spine and the pubic tubercle (Fig. 11.17). The needle is inserted 0.5 cm below the junction of the lateral third and medial two-thirds of the in-guinal ligament.

The needle is advanced in a sagittal plane at an angle of 60° to the skin, with the bevel of the needle parallel to the skin (Fig. 11.18). A syringe containing saline is attached to the needle

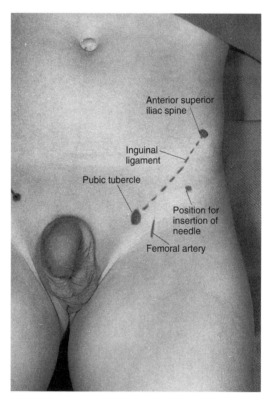

**Fig. 11.17**   Fascia iliaca block. The position of the left inguinal ligament is indicated by a line drawn between the anterior superior iliac spine and the pubic tubercle. The position of the femoral artery is marked.

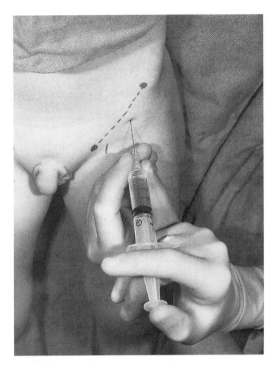

**Fig. 11.18**   Fascia iliaca block. The needle is inserted 0.5 cm below the junction of the lateral third and medial two-thirds of the inguinal ligament. The needle is advanced in a sagittal plane at an angle of 60° to the skin, with the bevel of the needle parallel to the skin.

and pressure gently applied to the barrel of the syringe as the needle is advanced. There is loss of resistance twice as the needle tip penetrates the fascia lata and fascia iliaca. The needle is then gently aspirated with a syringe before local anaesthetic is injected immediately deep to the fascia iliaca.

As the local anaesthetic is injected, pressure is applied immediately distal to the needle to encourage spread of the local anaesthetic into the fascia iliaca compartment (Fig. 11.19). After injection the local anaesthetic is massaged towards the inguinal ligament.

An 18 g cannula can be used to site a 20 g catheter within the fascia iliaca compartment (e.g. Contiplex® from B Braun Med Ltd or the brachial plexus set from Arrow® International, Inc.)

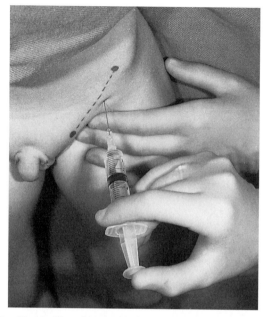

**Fig. 11.19**   Fascia iliaca block. As the local anaesthetic is injected, pressure is applied immediately distal to the needle to encourage spread of the local anaesthetic into the fascia iliaca compartment.

(Fig. 11.20). Once the needle has perforated the fascia iliaca the cannula is depressed towards the thigh. The cannula is advanced its full length over the needle which is then removed. A catheter is threaded 2–4 cm into the fascia iliaca compartment and the cannula withdrawn. The catheter is secured in a loop with a transparent dressing. Increments or continuous infusions of local anaesthetic can be given to prolong the duration of block.

## REFERENCES

Dalens, B., Vanneuville, G., and Tanguy, A. (1989). Comparison of the fascia iliaca compartment block with the 3-in-1 block in children. *Anesthesia Analgesia*, **69**, 705–13.

Winnie, A. P., Ramamurthy, S., and Durrani, Z. (1973). The inguinal paravascular technic of lumbar plexus anesthesia: the '3-in-1 block'. *Anesthesia Analgesia*, **52**, 989–96.

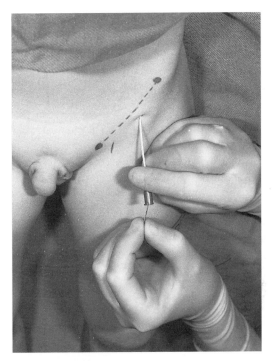

**Fig. 11.20**   Fascia iliaca block. An 18 g cannula can be used to site a 20 g catheter within the fascia iliaca compartment.

## NERVE BLOCKS AROUND THE KNEE AND ANKLE

The lower leg and foot are innervated by the saphenous nerve and the divisions of the sciatic nerve. These are easily blocked at the knee or ankle.

### The divisions of the sciatic nerve

The sciatic nerve divides in the lower third of the posterior thigh into the tibial and common peroneal nerves. These divisions cross the back of the knee within the popliteal fossa and together innervate most of the skin below the knee.

168 *J. M. Peutrell*

### The tibial nerve (L4–S3)

The sensory branches of the tibial nerve (Fig. 11.1) are:

(1) the sural nerve, which supplies the posterolateral aspect of the lower one-third of the leg, the lateral malleolus, and the outer borders of the foot and little toe;

(2) the medial calcaneal nerve, which perforates the flexor retinaculum at the ankle to supply the skin of the medial surface of the heel;

(3) the continuation of the tibial nerve, which passes behind the medial malleolus to divide into medial and lateral plantar branches and supplies the skin of the sole of the foot, the nail beds, the skin over the dorsal aspects of the terminal phalanges, and the joints of the tarsus and metatarsus;

(4) articular branches to the knee and ankle joints.

The motor branches of the tibial nerve innervate the flexors of the calf and foot and the muscles that invert the foot.

### The common peroneal nerve (L4–S2)

The sensory branches of the common peroneal nerve (Fig. 11.1) are:

(1) articular branches to the knee and superior tibio-fibular joint;

(2) the lateral cutaneous nerve of the calf, which supplies the lateral aspect of the upper half of the calf;

(3) the peroneal communicating branch, which joins the medial sural nerve to form the sural nerve supplying the skin of the posterolateral lower third of the leg;

(4) the deep peroneal nerve, which supplies a cutaneous branch to the interdigital cleft between the first and second toes, and articular branches to the ankle, tarsal, and the first to fourth metatarsophalangeal joints,

(5) the superficial peroneal nerve, which supplies the skin of the lower lateral leg, lateral malleolus, dorsum of foot and the interdigital clefts (except between the first and second toes).

Stimulation of the common peroneal nerve causes dorsiflexion of the foot and toes and eversion at the ankle.

## Saphenous nerve

The saphenous nerve is the largest cutaneous branch of the femoral nerve and supplies sensation to the medial lower leg and the foot, sometimes as far as the metatarsophalangeal joint of the big toe (Fig. 11.1).

# BLOCKADE OF THE TIBIAL AND COMMON PERONEAL NERVES WITHIN THE POPLITEAL FOSSA

*Anatomy*

The popliteal fossa is a diamond-shaped area at the back of the knee (Fig. 11.21). It is bordered above by the biceps femoris laterally and by the semimembranosus and semitendinosus medially, and below by the medial and lateral heads of the gastrocnemius. The popliteal fossa can be imagined as having upper and lower triangles (Fig. 11.21).

The tibial nerve crosses from the apex of the upper triangle to just lateral of the mid-point of the intercondylar line. The nerve lies lateral to the popliteal artery in the upper part of the fossa but then crosses the artery to lie on its medial side in the lower part.

The common peroneal nerve runs along the upper lateral border of the popliteal fossa close to biceps femoris and leaves the fossa by crossing superficial to the lateral head of the gastrocnemius.

Both tibial and common peroneal nerves lie deep to the popliteal membrane.

*Indications*

(1) Operations within the distribution of the nerves (e.g. correction of talipes);
(2) to facilitate physiotherapy in children with a spastic equinus foot deformity;
(3) as a diagnostic block in children with abnormal gait secondary to myotonia.

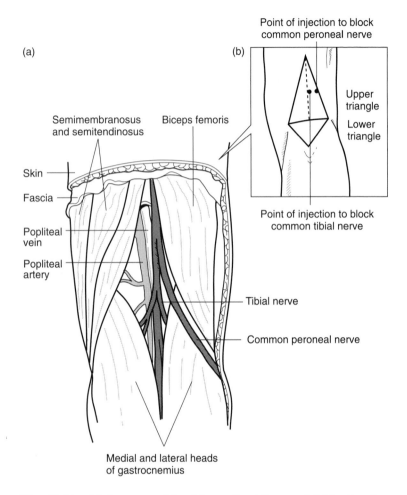

**Fig. 11.21** (a) Anatomy of the right popliteal fossa and (b) landmarks for blocks of the tibial and common peroneal nerves.

### Equipment

2.5 cm 22 or 24 g short-bevelled needle, peripheral nerve stimulator, tubing to connect the needle and syringe.

### Drugs

Bupivacaine 0.5 per cent in a total dose of 0.5 ml kg$^{-1}$.

## Complications

(1) Penetration of the popliteal artery which lies deep to the tibial nerve at the point of injection;
(2) (rarely) damage to the nerves producing dysaesthesia, hypoaesthesia, and footdrop.

## Technique

The boundaries of the upper triangle of the popliteal fossa are biceps femoris laterally, and semimembranosus and semitendinosus medially. The intercondylar line is indicated by the skin crease at the back of the knee. The position of the popliteal artery and the point of needle insertion for tibial nerve block (X) are marked (Fig. 11.22).

The child lies prone or semi-prone with the leg to be blocked uppermost. The skin over the back of the knee is cleaned with an alcoholic antiseptic solution.

### Tibial nerve block

A needle is inserted at right angles to the skin half-way between the intercondylar line and the apex of the upper triangle of the popliteal fossa, just lateral to the pulsations of the popliteal artery (Fig. 11.23). The risk of damage to the artery is reduced by using a peripheral nerve stimulator to find the tibial nerve. A 'pop' is felt as the needle penetrates the popliteal membrane. The tibial nerve lies about 0.5 cm deep to the membrane. Stimulation with the peripheral nerve stimulator causes plantar flexion and inversion of the foot. After aspiration local anaesthetic is injected.

### Common peroneal nerve block

The needle is inserted at the lateral border of the popliteal fossa at the same level as for tibial nerve block (Fig. 11.24). The needle is advanced at right angles to the skin and a 'pop' is felt as the needle penetrates the popliteal membrane. The nerve lies immediately below the membrane and stimulation with the peripheral nerve stimulator causes dorsiflexion and eversion of the foot. After aspiration local anaesthetic is injected.

## REFERENCES

Kempthorne, P. M. and Brown, T. C. K. (1984). Nerve blocks around the knee in children. *Anaesthesia Intensive Care*, **12**, 14–17.

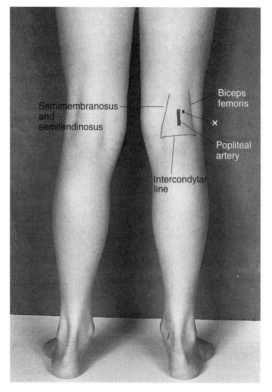

**Fig. 11.22**   Blockade of the tibial and common peroneal nerves within the popliteal fossa. The boundaries of the upper triangle of the popliteal fossa are biceps femoris laterally, and semimembranous and semitendinosus medially. The intercondylar line is indicated by the skin crease at the back of the knee. The position of the popliteal artery and the point of needle insertion for tibial nerve block (X) are marked.

## SAPHENOUS NERVE BLOCK

*Anatomy*

The saphenous nerve descends vertically along the medial side of the knee behind sartorius. It then emerges between the gracilis and sartorius and penetrates the deep fascia of the knee to lie subcutaneously (Fig. 11.25). The saphenous nerve descends in the lower leg behind the saphenous vein.

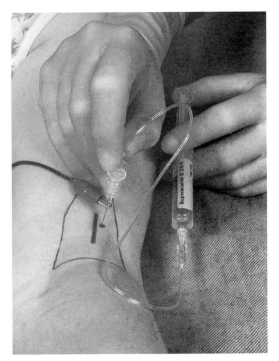

**Fig. 11.23**    Tibial nerve block.

*Indications*

For operations on the medial parts of the lower leg, ankle, and upper foot (often combined with blocks of the tibial and common peroneal nerves).

*Equipment*

25 g hypodermic needle.

*Drugs*

2–3 ml 0.5 per cent bupivacaine.

*Complications*

Penetration of the saphenous vein.

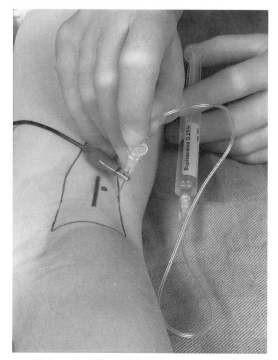

**Fig. 11.24**   Common peroneal nerve block.

## Technique

The saphenous nerve is blocked with a subcutaneous injection of local anaesthetic along the dotted line drawn from the medial part of the tibial tuberosity to the anterior border of the gastrocnemius muscle (Fig. 11.26).

## NERVE BLOCKS AROUND THE ANKLE

### Anatomy

The foot is supplied by five nerves (Fig. 11.1) which are easy to block at the ankle:

(1)   tibial;
(2)   sural;
(3)   superficial peroneal;

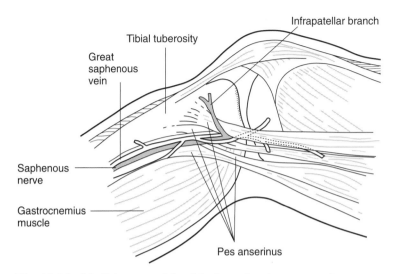

**Fig. 11.25**   Medial aspect of the right knee showing course of saphenous nerve.

(4)  deep peroneal; and
(5)  saphenous.

*The tibial nerve*

Passes behind the medial malleolus deep to the flexor retinaculum and immediately posterior to the posterior tibial artery (Fig. 11.27). It gives off three branches:

(1)  the medial calcaneal branch perforates the flexor retinaculum to supply the skin of the medial heel;
(2)  the medial plantar nerve supplies the skin of the medial two-thirds of the sole of the foot and the plantar surface of the medial three and a half toes;
(3)  the lateral plantar nerve supplies the skin of the lateral one-third of the sole of the foot and the plantar surface of the lateral one and a half toes.

*The sural nerve*

Arises from the union of a branch of the tibial nerve with a branch of the common peroneal nerve. It passes below and behind the

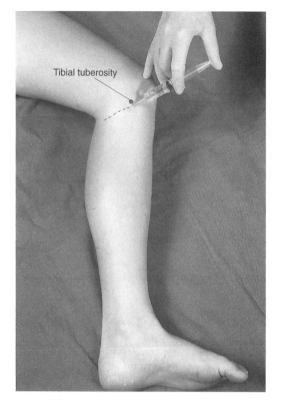

**Fig. 11.26** Saphenous nerve block.

lateral malleolus midway between the malleolus and the cal-
caneum, accompanied by the short saphenous vein. It supplies
sensation to the skin of the lateral surface of the foot and little toe.

*Superficial peroneal nerve*

This perforates the deep fascia on the anterior surface of the distal
two-thirds of the lower leg to run in the superficial fascia over the
lateral half of the ankle and the dorsum of the foot (Fig. 11.28). It
supplies the skin of the dorsum of the foot and toes except the
cleft between the first and second toes.

*Deep peroneal nerve*

This descends the anterior lower leg lying on the interosseus
membrane. It passes beneath the extensor retinaculum to enter

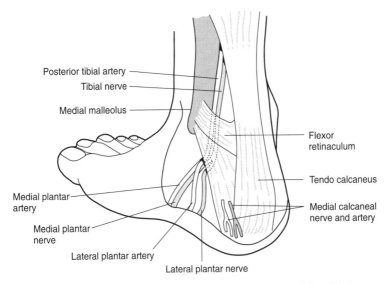

**Fig. 11.27**   The medial malleolus, showing the course of the tibial nerve.

the foot half-way between the medial and lateral malleolus. In the upper foot the deep peroneal nerve lies lateral to the anterior tibial artery and the tendon of the extensor hallucis longus muscle. It supplies the skin of the cleft between the first and second toes and articular branches to the joints of the foot (Fig. 11.28).

*Saphenous nerve*
Descends in the lower leg behind the great saphenous vein to run subcutaneously in front of the medial malleolus (Fig. 11.28). It supplies the skin of the medial malleolus and the medial part of the proximal foot, sometimes as far as the metatarsophalangeal joints.

*Indications*
Operations on the foot or toes.

*Equipment*
23 g hypodermic needle.

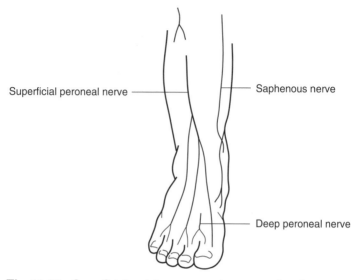

**Fig. 11.28** Superficial and deep peroneal nerves and saphenous nerve in the foot.

### Drugs

Bupivacaine 0.5 per cent 1–5 ml per nerve (in a total dose not exceeding 2.5 mg kg$^{-1}$ bupivacaine).

### Duration of action

3–4 hours.

### Complications

Complications potentially include neuropraxia. Intravascular injection of local anaesthetic is unlikely.

### Technique

#### Tibial nerve block

The skin over the medial ankle is cleaned with an alcoholic antiseptic solution. The needle is inserted at right angles to the skin

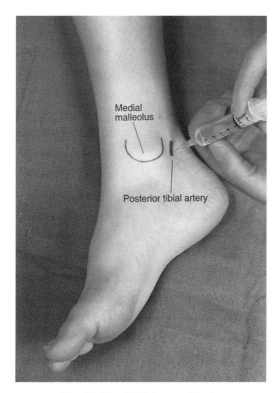

**Fig. 11.29**   Tibial nerve block.

immediately behind the pulsations of the posterior tibial artery
(Fig. 11.29). If the pulsations of the artery cannot be felt, then the
needle is inserted at the level of the upper border of the medial
malleolus half-way between the Achilles tendon and the medial
malleolus. Local anaesthetic is injected at a depth midway
between skin and bone.

*Sural nerve block*

The skin over the lower leg and upper foot is cleaned with an
alcoholic antiseptic solution. The needle is inserted midway
between the posterior border of the lateral malleolus and the posterior border of the calcaneus (Fig. 11.30). A subcutaneous wheal
that expands the space between the lateral malleolus and the
Achilles tendon is raised.

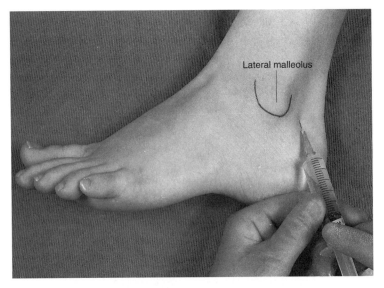

**Fig. 11.30**   Sural nerve block.

*Superficial peroneal nerve block*
Local anaesthetic is injected subcutaneously in a line between the lateral malleolus and the anterior border of the tibia (Fig. 11.31).

*Deep peroneal nerve block*
The nerve is blocked just above the level of the malleoli lateral to the tendon of extensor hallucis longus and immediately lateral to the pulsations of the anterior tibial artery (Fig. 11.32). The needle is inserted at right angles to the skin and local anaesthetic is injected deep to the extensor retinaculum of the ankle joint.

*Saphenous nerve block*
Local anaesthetic is infiltrated subcutaneously in a line between the upper level of the medial malleolus and the anterior border of the tibia (Fig. 11.33). In practice the superficial peroneal and saphenous nerves are blocked with a single subcutaneous injection of local anaesthetic running from the medial to lateral malleoli.

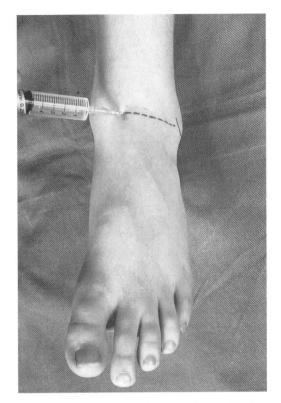

**Fig. 11.31**   Superficial peroneal nerve block.

## METATARSAL BLOCKS

The main advantage of metatarsal block is that there is less distortion of the structures of the toe during surgery because local anaesthetic is injected more proximally than with a ring block of the toes.

### *Anatomy*

The plantar digital nerves run on either side of the metatarsal bones to supply the joints of the toes, the structures around the nails, and the skin of all but the dorsal surface of the toes. There are three common digital nerves supplying the adjacent sides of the first and second, second and third, and third and fourth toes. The medial side of the big toe is supplied by a branch of the

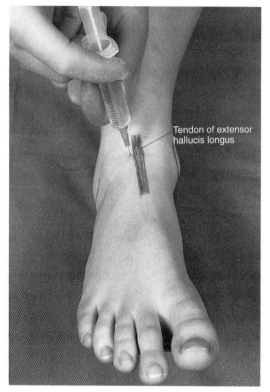

Tendon of extensor
hallucis longus

**Fig. 11.32**   Deep peroneal nerve block.

medial plantar nerve and the little toe is supplied by a superficial
branch of the lateral plantar nerve and the sural nerve.

### Indications
Operations on the toes (e.g. removal of nail, tendon transfer).

### Equipment
23 g hypodermic needle.

### Drugs
Bupivacaine 0.5 per cent 1–2 ml (depending on the size of the
child), injected on either side of the metatarsal bones. *Local anaes-*

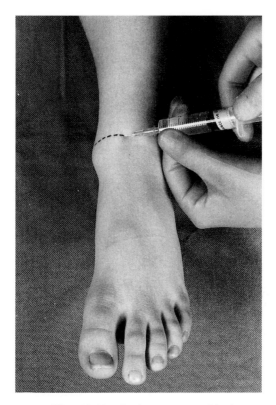

**Fig. 11.33**   Saphenous nerve block.

*thetic solutions containing adrenaline should never be used because of
the risk of gangrene of the toes.*

## Technique

The skin over the extensor surface of the lower foot is cleaned
with an alcoholic antiseptic solution. The needle is inserted
through the extensor surface of the foot on the lateral side of the
base of the metatarsal bone. The needle is advanced until it can
be felt through the sole of the foot taking care not to pierce the
skin of the sole (Fig. 11.34). After aspiration local anaesthetic is
injected in a volume sufficient to produce a palpable swelling.
The dorsal digital nerves are blocked by injecting local anaesthetic

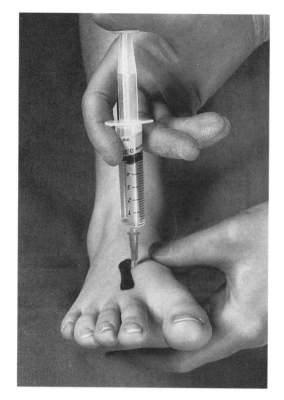

**Fig. 11.34**   Metatarsal block.

subcutaneously as the needle is withdrawn. The injection is repeated on the medial side of the metatarsal bone.

# Part 4

# Techniques of regional anaesthesia: neuraxial anaesthesia

# 12

## Extradural anaesthesia

J. M. PEUTRELL

### THORACIC EXTRADURAL ANAESTHESIA

Extradural catheters are rarely inserted at the thoracic level in children. The depth of the extradural space and distance between the tissues planes is smaller and the potential for spinal cord damage and dural puncture is probably greater than in adults. Thoracic extradurals are difficult to insert in awake children and damage to the spinal cord by the extradural needle will not be recognized in anaesthetized children. Analgesia for thoracic dermatomes can usually be obtained using an extradural block inserted at the lumbar level (see below).

There are few indications for using a thoracic approach to the extradural space and the technique should be used only by experienced anaesthetists. It will not be described further.

### LUMBAR EXTRADURAL ANAESTHESIA

*Anatomy*

In full-term babies, the spinal cord extends to L3 and the dura to S3 or S4. During the first year of life the vertebral column grows faster than the spinal cord, and by 12 months of age the terminations of the dura and spinal cord are in the adult position: the dura finishes at the S2 and the spinal cord at the L1 or L2 vertebrae. The sacrum of children lies higher relative to the iliac crests than in adults. In neonates the intercristal line indicates the position of L5–S1 and in children the position of L5.

During childhood the sacrum is incompletely ossified and the sacral vertebral bodies are separate. Fusion of the sacral vertebrae

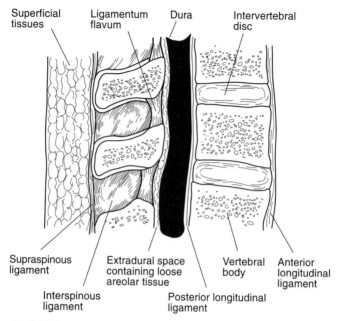

**Fig. 12.1**   Diagram showing the lumbar vertebral column in sagittal section.

begins at about 18 years of age at S4 and S5 and then extends upwards. Fusion of the sacrum is not complete until 25–30 years of age. Extradural needles can, therefore, be inserted through the sacral intervertebral spaces in childhood. The S2–S3 interspace is the largest and easiest to identify and lies just below the termination of the dura in children older than 12 months. A line drawn between the posterior superior iliac spin crosses the arch of the second sacral vertebra.

The extradural space is filled with loose areolar tissue which becomes more densely packed in children older than 8 years. Local anaesthetics spread extensively and extradural catheters are easy to thread. The tip of an extradural catheter can usually be positioned at the thoracic level using a lumbar or caudal approach. A sagittal view of the lumbar spine is shown in Fig. 12.1.

The resistance of the interspinous ligaments and ligamentum flavum in children is much less compared with adults. The depth of the extradural space in children older than neonates correlates with age and weight but there is significant variability between patients (Fig. 12.2): it can be as little as 4 mm in a neonate or 10 mm in a 4-year-old. The approximate depth of the extradural space is given by the equations shown in Table 12.1.

The depth of the lumbar epidural space in neonates is about 10 mm (range: 4–15 mm) (Hasan *et al.* 1994).

### Indications

Lumbar extradural analgesia can be used in children heavier than about 5 kg having operations on the lower abdomen or leg.

A catheter inserted at the lumbar level can also be used to obtain analgesia within thoracic dermatomes by:

(1)  advancing the catheter a little further cephalad;
(2)  using a larger volume of local anaesthetic;
(3)  injecting opioids into the extradural space.

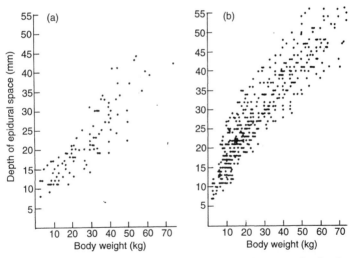

**Fig. 12.2**  Nomograms showing the relationship between the depth of the extradural space and body weight at (a) the sacral and (b) lumbar levels. (From Dalens, B. O. and Chrysostome, Y. (1991). Intervertebral epidural anaesthesia in paediatric surgery: success rate and adverse effects in 650 consecutive procedures. *Paediatric Anaesthesia*, **1**, 107–17, with kind permission.)

**Table 12.1** Depth of extradural space in children at different vertebral levels calculated according to (a) age and (b) body weight

| Author | Vertebral level | Calculation |
|---|---|---|
| (a) | | |
| Busoni (1990) | L2–L3 | $(2 \times$ age in years$) + 10$ (mm) |
| Hasan *et al.* (1994) | Lumbar | $1 + (0.15 \times$ age in years$)$ (cm) |
| (b) | | |
| Uemura and Yamashita (1992) | L3–L4 | (body weight in kg $+ 10) \times 0.8$ (mm) |
| Hasan *et al.* (1994) | Lumbar | $0.8 + (0.05 \times$ body weight in kg$)$ (cm) |

A lumbar extradural catheter can therefore be used to provide analgesia for:

(1) thoracotomy;
(2) upper abdominal incisions;
(3) fractured ribs.

A catheter technique has two advantages compared with a single injection of local anaesthetic into the caudal extradural space:

(1) for operations in the thoraco-lumbar dermatomes, the dose of local anaesthetic is reduced because it can be injected at the appropriate segmental level;
(2) further local anaesthetic can be injected through the catheter to prolong the duration of analgesia during surgery or to provide postoperative pain relief.

A catheter inserted at the lumbar level is less likely than one inserted through the sacral hiatus to become contaminated with faecal bacteria.

## Contraindications

(1) local infection;
(2) septicaemia;
(3) coagulopathy;
(4) raised intracranial pressure or hydrocephalus;
(5) meningomyelocoele or spina bifida;

(6) vertebral implants (e.g. Harrington rods), unless placed under direct vision at operation;
(7) local neurological disease;
(8) uncorrected hypovolaemia.

## Equipment

### Extradural needles

Catheters are usually inserted into the lumbar extradural space through a Tuohy needle (Table 12.2 and Fig. 1.6). A Tuohy needle has a contoured end designed to direct the catheter along the extradural space and reduce the risk of dural puncture. It also has a solid stylet to prevent implanting skin into the extradural space. Tuohy needles are manufactured in various sizes for use in children of different weights:

(1) 17 or 18 g needles, 8 or 9 cm long, marked at 1 cm intervals, suitable for children weighing more than 25 kg;
(2) 19 g needles, 5 cm long, marked at 0.5 cm intervals, used in children weighing less than 25 kg.

### Extradural catheters

22–24 g catheters marked at 0.5 or 1 cm intervals are used in small children. In older children, 18 and 19 g catheters marked at 1 cm intervals are suitable. Smaller catheters usually have a single end-hole and the larger catheters either an end-hole or three lateral eyes.

## Drugs

The spread of local anaesthetic is less predictable in the lumbar and thoracic than the caudal extradural space: spread is more extensive the higher the local anaesthetic is injected and is greater in a rostral than caudal direction. The spread in the thoracic extradural space is approximately 50 per cent more than within the caudal space.

Various schemes are used to calculate the volume of local anaesthetic needed to obtain adequate analgesia:

1. The volume of local anaesthetic injected into the caudal extradural space is $(0.056 \text{ ml kg}^{-1}) \times$ (number of segments to be blocked) (Takasaki *et al.* 1977). This formula is often used

**Table 12.2** Some extradural needles and catheters suitable for use in children

| Manufacturer | Tuohy needle | | | Gauge | Extradural catheter | | |
|---|---|---|---|---|---|---|---|
| | Length cm | Gauge | Interval marks (cm) | | Distal/end holes | Interval marks (cm) | Material |
| Portex Ltd | 5 | 19 | 0.5 | 23 | Single end | 1.0 (from 5 to 15 cm) | Nylon |
| | 8 | 18 | 1.0 | 18 | Single end or three lateral eyes | 1.0 (from 5 to 15 cm) | Nylon |
| Vygon UK Ltd | 5 | 19 | 0.5 | 22 | Single end | 0.5 (thro'out) (distal 20 cm) | Polyurethane |
| | 9 | 17 | 1.0 | 19 | Single end | 1.0 (from 5 to 20 cm) | Polyethylene (with stylet) |
| | 9 | 17 | 1.0 | 19 | Single end or three lateral eyes | 1.0 (from 5 to 20 cm) | Polyurethrane |

to calculate the volume needed when local anaesthetic is injected at lumbar level.

2. The initial volume of 0.25 per cent bupivacaine for lumbar extradural analgesia for operations on the abdomen or leg is (Murat *et al.* 1987):
   < 20 kg body weight: 0.75 ml kg$^{-1}$
   > 100 cm height: 0.1 ml cm$^{-1}$.
3. An initial volume of 0.5 ml kg$^{-1}$ of 0.25 per cent bupivacaine with a subsequent infusion of 0.08 ml kg$^{-1}$ is suitable for lumbar extradural analgesia for operations on the genitalia or leg (Desparmet *et al.* 1990).

To reduce the risk of systemic toxicity, the initial dose of bupivacaine should not exceed 2.5 mg kg$^{-1}$ and the subsequent doses should be less than 0.5 mg kg$^{-1}$ h$^{-1}$.

Adrenaline, 1 : 200 000 prolongs the duration of action of bupivacaine in children younger than 8 years of age but has been implicated in spinal cord infarction in babies having a continuous infusion.

*Technique of injection of local anaesthetic and the use of a test dose*

Intravascular placement of a catheter may not be recognized despite a test aspiration for two probable reasons:

(1) blood does not flow easily through epidural catheters of narrow bore;

(2) the pressure within epidural veins may be less than right atrial pressure when the child is in the lateral position and aspiration may simply collapse the vessel walls and not draw blood along the catheter.

Some authors recommend using a test dose of 0.5 $\mu$g kg$^{-1}$ of adrenaline while monitoring the arterial blood pressure, ECG, and heart rate. This is equivalent to 0.1 ml kg$^{-1}$ of a local anaesthetic solution containing 1 : 200 000 adrenaline. The injection is assumed to be intravascular if there is a significant increase in heart rate or blood pressure and no arrhythmias. However, in children anaesthetized with halothane the test dose may be unreliable. Adrenaline 0.5 $\mu$g kg$^{-1}$ injected intravenously produces a rise in blood pressure lasting less than 60 seconds and an increase in heart rate of only about 10 beats per minute. In some children this dose produces no significant increase in heart rate and a negative test dose will not exclude intravascular injection.

To reduce the risk of toxicity the following additional precautions should be taken:

(1)  aspirate the catheter gently before injecting local anaesthetic, and repeatly during the injection;
(2)  inject the local anaesthetic slowly (over 5–10 minutes) to reduce the peak concentration. The risk of toxic side-effects correlates with the peak concentration and the peak concentration for a given dose of local anaesthetic depends on the rate of injection.

## Complications

### Puncture of the dura

The rate of dural puncture by experienced anaesthetists is 0–2 per cent. It is higher if a 'loss of resistance' technique using saline instead of air is employed or relatively large extradural needles are used in small children.

Puncture of the dura can cause:

1.  A total spinal block. A large volume of local anaesthetic injected into the subarachnoid space will produce a sudden, total spinal block. The signs include:

    (a)  decreased ventilatory rate and apnoea;
    (b)  dilated pupils;
    (c)  loss of conciousness;
    (d)  hypotension in older children.

    Treatment of a total spinal block includes:

    (a)  intubation of the trachea and positive pressure ventilation of the lungs;
    (b)  support of the circulation of older children using intravenous fluids and vasopressor drugs. Severe hypotension is not usually a feature in children younger than 6 years.

    Surgery can continue once treatment of the total spinal block has been initiated and if the child is haemodynamically stable. The block usually persists for a couple of hours.

2.  A dural puncture headache. The incidence of post-lumbar-puncture headache in children is low. The clinical features include: postural headache, photophobia, nausea, and vomiting. Intractable headache can be treated with an autologous blood patch (5–10 ml).

*Subdural placement of the catheter*
This produces an unexpectedly high block of slower onset than a total spinal block.

*Vascular trauma*
Blood is aspirated from the extradural needle in about 1 per cent of children. The risk of penetration of an extradural vessel may be increased if extradural vessels are distended by positive pressure ventilation of the lungs or if a large-gauge Tuohy needle is used. Trauma to blood vesels may be complicated by:

(1) inadvertent injection of local anaesthetic into the circulation, causing convulsions and cardiac toxicity;
(2) venous or paradoxical arterial air emboli. Air is a sensitive indicator for loss of resistance within the extradural space. Large volumes should NEVER be injected deliberately because of the risk of venous air embolus if an extradural vessel has been punctured. The minimum volume of air that will produce significant cardiovascular depression when injected into a vein in humans is unknown. A very small volume could have serious consequences if there is a paradoxical embolus (e.g. across a patent foramen ovale). Carbon dioxide can be used instead of air to minimize this risk. Sterile saline can be used to test for loss of resistance but is much less sensitive and may dilute local anaesthetic solutions;
(3) extradural haematoma (rare).

*Migration of catheters*
Migration of catheters into the subdural or subarachnoid spaces or vessels occurs rarely during continuous extradural analgesia, producing either a high block or systemic toxicity.

*Hypotension*
This is very uncommon in children younger than 6 years of age. The haemodynamic stability observed in young children may be due to:

(1) a lower sympathetic tone compared with adults that is little affected by further sympathetic block;
(2) reduced blood volume within the lower limbs;
(3) compensatory vasoconstriction in the arms.

*Trauma to nerves*

The tips of catheters occasionally impinge against nerve roots. To reduce the risks of nerve damage a catheter should not be advanced forcibly against an obstruction.

*Infection*

Infection causing meningitis or extradural abcess is rare.

*Urinary retention*

This is uncommon if opioids are not used.

*Knotting, kinking, or breakage of the catheter*

Catheters can shear at points of weakness (e.g. at the side holes) or if they are pulled back through an extradural needle. The greater the amount of catheter threaded, the greater the risk of knotting of the catheter. It is generally recommended that broken catheters are not removed surgically.

## Difficulties

*Difficulty threading the catheter*

This occurs more commonly with fine catheters and is often attributed to the catheter tip impinging against one of the following:

(1)  mid-line fibrous septa dividing the dorsal compartment of the extradural space;
(2)  the inferior border of the lamina of a vertebra;
(3)  a nerve root.

The catheter should never be advanced forcibly against an obstruction because of the risk of nerve damage. An obstruction can sometimes be overcome by gently flexing or extending the child's back within the normal range of movement.

*Failure to locate the extradural space*

The extradural space cannot be found in about 5 per cent of children.

*Unilateral block*

This occurs in about 1 per cent of lumbar extradurals in children and is usually attributed to fibrous mid-line bands. The block on either side differs by more than three dermatomes in about 5 per cent of children and is higher on the side that was dependent when the extradural block was inserted.

### Patchy block

This is usually attributed to air bubbles within the extradural space interefering with the uptake of local anaesthetic into nerves. It occurs in about 4 per cent of children in whom air is used to test for loss of resistance, but the distribution of affected nerves is often outside the site of incision. Carbon dioxide can be used to test for 'loss of resistance' and is not associated with a patchy block.

### Technique

Extradural catheters are usually inserted in anaesthetised children. An intravenous cannula is sited and the blood pressure and electrocardiograph monitored. The child is turned onto the left side with the hips flexed (Fig. 12.3).

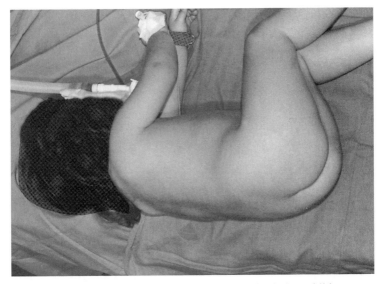

**Fig. 12.3**   Position for lumbar extradural anaesthesia in a child.

The position of the right iliac crest and the spinous processes of the fourth and fifth lumbar and first sacral vertebrae are shown (Fig. 12.4). The intercristal line crosses L5 in the mid-line. The skin over the lower back and buttocks is cleaned with an alcoholic antiseptic solution.

The index finger of the left hand palpates the interspinous space below the termination of the spinal cord, with the second finger and thumb lying either side of the mid-line. A 'nick' is made in the skin and the extradural needle with stylet is inserted (with the bevel facing cranially) in the mid-line half-way between the spinous processes (Fig. 12.5). The intervertebral spaces of L3–L4, L4–L5, L5–S1, S1–S2 or S2–S3 can be used in babies. The L2–L3 can also be used in older children. The needle is advanced at 90° to the skin in babies and about 80° in a rostral direction in children.

As the needle is advanced its tip passes through skin, subcutaneous tissues, and the supraspinous ligament. Once the needle is 'gripped' by the ligament the stylette is removed and a 10 ml loss of resistance syringe containing air is carefully attached. The back of the left hand of the anaesthetist is laid against the child's back, holding the hub of the extradural needle between the index and second fingers to control the needle as it is advanced (Fig. 12.6).

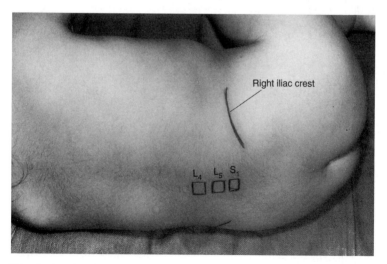

**Fig. 12.4**  Landmarks for lumbar extradural anaesthesia in a child.

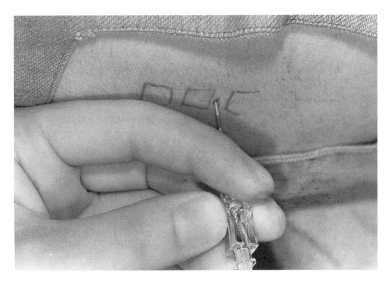

**Fig. 12.5**   The extradural needle is inserted in the mid-line half-way between the spinous processes.

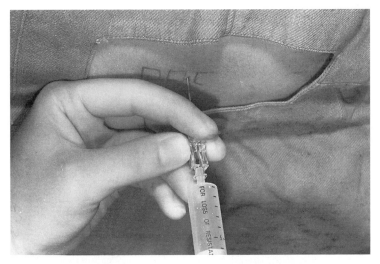

**Fig. 12.6**   The needle is carefully advanced at 90° in babies and 80° in a rostral direction in children. A loss of resistance syringe containing air or saline is used to identify the extradural space.

The needle is advanced carefully only a fraction of a millimetre and 'loss of resistance' tested for by lightly pressing the barrel of the syringe with the thumb of the right hand. To reduce the risk of air embolism, air should not be deliberately injected into the extradural space. The needle tip passes through the supraspinous and interspinous ligaments and the ligamentum flavum. The depth of the extradural space is short, and the resistance of the interspinous ligament and ligamentum flavum much weaker than in adults. A marked increase in tissue resistance when passing through the ligamentum flavum is not always found.

Once the extradural space is located, the syringe is removed and the catheter threaded 1.5–2 cm into the extradural space (Fig. 12.7). If analgesia within thoracic dermatomes is required, the catheter is threaded the distance between the site of entry and the desired segmental level. The catheters usually thread easily because the extradural fat is so loose.

While holding the catheter close to the hub of the needle, the needle is carefully removed, taking care not to pull out the catheter. The catheter is then secured securely in a double loop with a transparent dressing and taped to the child's back. The open end of the catheter is gently aspirated with a syringe and the

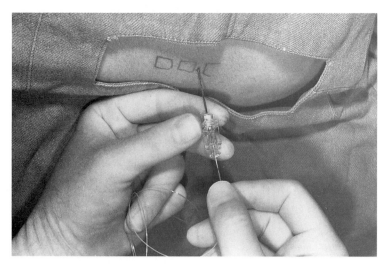

**Fig. 12.7** Once the extradural space is located, the catheter is threaded 1.5–2 cm in the extradural space.

lumen of the catheter examined for cerebrospinal fluid and blood. A 0.2 μm filter flushed with local anaesthetic is then attached to the catheter. Local anaesthetic is injected in a volume according to the child's weight and the number of segments to be blocked.

## FURTHER READING

Dalens, B. (1989). Regional anesthesia in children. *Anesthesia Analgesia*, **68**, 654–72.

Goldman, L. J. (1995). Complications in regional anaesthesia (editorial). *Paediatric Anaesthesia*, **5**, 3–9.

Yaster, M. and Maxwell, L. G. (1989). Pediatric regional anesthesia. *Anesthesiology*, **70**, 324–38.

## REFERENCES

Berde, C. B. (1992). Convulsions associated with pediatric regional anesthesia. *Anesthesia Analgesia*, **75**, 164–6.

Busoni, P. (1990). Anatomy. In *Regional anaesthesia in children*, (ed. C. Saint-Maurice and O. Schulte-Steinberg), pp. 16–25. Appleton & Lange/Mediglobe, Norwalk, San Mateo, Fribourg.

Busoni, P. and Messeri, A. (1989). Spinal anesthesia in children: surface anatomy. *Anesthesia Analgesia*, **68**, 418–19.

Busoni, P. and Sarti, A. (1987). Sacral intervertebral epidural block. *Anesthesiology*, **67**, 993–5.

Dalens, B. (1989). Regional anesthesia in children. *Anesthesia Analgesia*, **68**, 654–72.

Dalens, B. and Chrysostome, Y. (1991). Intervertebral epidural anaesthesia in paediatric surgery: success rate and adverse effects in 650 consecutive procedures. *Paediatric Anaesthesia*, **1**, 107–17.

Desparmet, J., Mateo, J., Ecoffey, C., and Mazoit, X. (1990). Efficacy of an epidural test dose in children anesthetised with halothane. *Anesthesiology*, **72**, 249–51.

Ghia, J. N., Spielman, F. J., and Stieber, S. F. (1984). The diagnosis and successful treatment of post-lumbar puncture headache in a pediatric patient. *Regional Anesthesia*, **9**, 102–5.

Hasan, M. A., Howard, R. F., and Lloyd-Thomas, R. (1994). Depth of epidural space in children. *Anaesthesia*, **49**, 1085–7.

Murat, I., Delleur, M. M., Esteve, C., Egu, J. F., Raynaud, P., and Saint-Maurice, C. (1987). Continuous extradural anaesthesia in children. *British Journal of Anaesthesia*, **69**, 1441–50.

Sethna, N. F. and Berde, C. B. (1993). Venous air embolism during identification of the epidural space in children. *Anesthesia Analgesia*, **76**, 925–7.

Takasaki, M., Dohi, S., Kawabata, Y., and Takahashi, T. (1977). Dosage of lidocaine for caudal anesthesia in infants and children. *Anesthesiology*, **47**, 527–9.

Uemura, A. and Yamashita, M. (1992). A formula for determining the distance from the skin to the lumbar epidural space in infants and children. *Paediatric Anaesthesia*, **2**, 305–7.

# CAUDAL EXTRADURAL ANAESTHESIA

## Anatomy

The sacrum is a triangular bone formed by the five sacral vertebrae. In childhood, the individual vertebrae are separated by cartilage and complete ossification of the sacrum does not occur until 20–30 years of age. The sacrum in a baby is relatively flat compared with older children and adults, in whom it is concave anteriorly (Fig. 12.8).

The sacral canal is formed by the laminae, pedicles, and bodies of the sacral vertebrae and contains the caudal extradural space, the cauda equina, the filum terminale, and the dura (ending at S2 in children and S3 in babies).

The caudal extradural space can be entered through the sacral hiatus. The sacral hiatus is formed by incomplete fusion of the fifth sacral vertebra and is covered by the dorsal sacrococcygeal ligaments, subcutaneous fat, and skin. With increasing age the size of the sacral hiatus decreases and by adulthood is sometimes completely calcified. The caudal extradural space of young children contains loose fatty tissue, allowing relatively easy spread of local anaesthetic solutions.

The position of the sacral hiatus can be found by one of three methods. The sacral hiatus lies:

(1)  as a concave depression between the sacral cornua above the sacrococcygeal joint;

(2)  at the apex of an equilateral triangle formed by the posterior superior iliac spines; and

(3)  in the mid-line at the end of a line drawn through the middle of the lateral thigh when the legs are flexed at the hips.

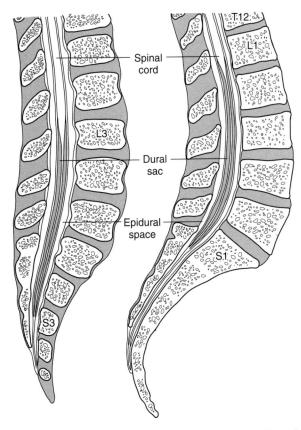

**Fig. 12.8** Saggital section of the sacrum in neonates (left) and adults (right).

## Indications

Caudal extradural anaesthesia is usually combined with light general anaesthesia to provide analgesia lasting 4–6 hours. The technique is particularly useful for operations on:

(1) the lower abdomen and perineum (e.g. inguinal herniotomy, orchidopexy, and operations on the bladder);

(2) the penis—especially for proximal hypospadias repair in which block of the dorsal penile nerves will not provide analgesia of the proximal penis (see Chapter 10, p. 132), circumcision.

(3)  operations on the legs (e.g. osteotomy of the hip, correction
     of talipes).

The technique is also used in awake babies having minor lower
abdominal operations who are at risk of postoperative apnoea.

### Contraindications
(1)  Local sepsis;
(2)  septicaemia;
(3)  coagulopathy;
(4)  active neurological disease;
(5)  meningomyelocoele;
(6)  hydrocephalus or raised intracranial pressure;
(7)  uncorrected hypotension;
(8)  major abnormalities of the sacrum.

### Equipment

*Needles*

Standard cutting needles are used by some anaesthetists but have
several disadvantages:

(1)  the 'pop' felt as the sacrococcygeal membrane is perforated is
     less easily appreciated;
(2)  cartilage and bone are more easily penetrated;
(3)  there is a higher incidence of penetration of blood vessels;
(4)  more of the needle must be advanced to ensure that all of the
     bevel lies within the sacral canal;
(5)  these needles do not have a stylet and there is a theoretical
     risk of causing an implantation dermoid.

Shorter-bevelled needles are associated with fewer complications
and give a more sensitive appreciation of changes in tissue resistance. Lumbar puncture needles have stylets and shorter bevels
and short versions can be used for caudal block.

Intravenous cannulae (e.g. 18 g or 20 g) are alternatives. The
needle acts as a stylet and the shoulders of the cannula give a
positive 'feel' as they penetrate the sacrococcygeal membrane.

The cannula can be advanced 1–2 cm over the needle with a relatively low risk of puncturing the dura or blood vessels, and local anaesthetic can be delivered through the cannula at a higher segmental level. If the cannula cannot be advanced easily, it unlikely that it lies within the caudal extradural space.

*Filter needles*

A filter needle should be used to draw up local anaesthetic to prevent the injection of glass particles into the extradural space.

### Drugs

The spread of local anaesthetic injected into the caudal extradural space in children less than about 7 years of age is predictable and correlates with age and weight. The volume of local anaesthetic can be obtained from formulae or nomograms:

(1)   the volume of local anaesthetic = 0.056 ml × body weight (in kg) × number of spinal segments to be blocked (Takasaki *et al.* 1977);

(2)   nomograms correlate the volume of local anaesthetic with the number of spinal segments to be blocked and with the ages and weights of children (Fig. 12.9).

The sensory block produced is usually within two dermatomes of the predicted level and the calculated volume of local anaesthetic injected should include two dermatomes above the desired level. Spread of local anaesthetic becomes much more unpredictable in children older than 7 years.

A popular and more simple scheme is described by Armitage (1989). Bupivacaine 0.25 per cent without adrenaline is injected in a volume according to weight and the site of operation (Table 12.3). Peak plasma concentrations of bupivacaine after injection of 3 mg kg$^{-1}$ into the caudal extradural space are less than 2 $\mu$g ml$^{-1}$ in children older than 4 months (Eyres *et al.* 1983).

If the dose of local anaesthetic predicted from these schemes is more than the maximum accepted dose, either:

(1)   a more dilute solution of local anaesthetic in the same volume can be injected; or

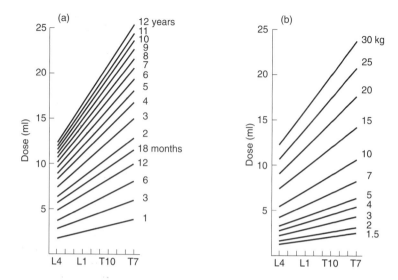

**Fig. 12.9** Nomograms showing the relationship between the spread of local anaesthetics from the caudal extradural space to different segmental levels with (a) age and (b) weight. The upper level of the block in dermatomes is shown on the *x* axis and the volume of local anaesthetic in millilitres is shown on the *y* axis. (From figure 1 in Busoni, P. and Andreucetti, T. (1986). The spread of caudal analgesia in children: a mathematical model. *Anaesthesia Intensive Care*, **14**, 140–4 with kind permission.)

**Table 12.3** Scheme described by Armitage (1989) for caudal anaesthesia using 0.25 per cent bupivacaine without adrenaline in children. Bupivacaine 0.19 per cent is used for volumes in excess of 20 ml (one part 0.9 per cent sodium chloride plus three parts 0.25 per cent bupivacaine).

| Segmental level of operation | dose (ml kg⁻¹) |
| --- | --- |
| Lumbo-sacral | 0.5 |
| Thoraco-lumbar | 1.0 |
| Mid-thoracic | 1.25 |

(2)  a cannula or catheter can be inserted into the sacral canal and used to deliver local anaesthetic at a higher segmental level; or
(3)  lumbar extradural anaesthesia can be used instead.

A single injection of local anaesthetic given into the caudal extradural space is rarely used to block the mid-thoracic dermatomes because of the large dose needed and the risk of systemic toxicity. Lumbar extradural analgesia is more widely used to provide analgesia for upper abdominal and thoracic surgery.

Bupivacaine 0.125 per cent produces analgesia similar to bupivacaine 0.25 per cent but with a significantly lower incidence of motor weakness. Bupivacaine 0.125 per cent is probably the solution of choice for most operations.

Lignocaine has a shorter duration of analgesia compared with bupivacaine.

### Duration of action

The duration of analgesia depends on:

(1)　the local anaesthetic used;
(2)　the dose of local anaesthetic;
(3)　sensory level of operation: the duration of analgesia is longer for operations in the lumbo-sacral dermatomes compared with thoraco-lumbar dermatomes when an equal volume and concentration of local anaesthetic is injected;
(4)　adrenaline significantly prolongs the duration of action of bupivacaine in children. The effects are inversely related to age and are most marked in children younger than 5 years.

Bupivacaine (0.125 and 0.25 per cent) with 1 : 200 000 adrenaline 0.75 ml kg$^{-1}$ produces analgesia lasting longer than 5 hours in 70 per cent of children having superficial lower abdominal and penile surgery (Wolf *et al.* 1988). The duration of analgesia may, however, be much shorter in babies.

### Onset of block

10–15 minutes.

### Failure rate

Caudal anaesthesia is easier in children younger than 7 years old compared with older children. Inadequate block can be caused by:

1.　Failure to penetrate the sacral hiatus. This is more common in children older than 7 years. Local anaesthetic may be injected

subcutaneously and obliterate the landmarks of the sacral hiatus. Subcutaneous injection is the most common cause of failed block.
2. Unilateral block. The level of block is often 1–2 dermatomes higher on the side that was dependent during the caudal injection. The incidence of complete unilateral block is about 2 per cent and is probably caused by mid-line extradural septa.
3. Missed segments. These are very uncommon and may be caused by air bubbles introduced into the caudal extradural space if loss of resistance to air is used to identify the caudal extradural space.

## Complications

### Intravascular injection

Intravascular injection of local anaesthetic may produce systemic toxicity if the peak plasma concentrations produced are within the toxic range (> 2–4 $\mu$g ml$^{-1}$). Peak concentrations are lower if drugs are injected slowly. Extradural veins have no valves and local anaesthetics can enter the cerebral circulation by retrograde flow, producing convulsions at a lower dose.

### Intraosseous injection

An intraosseous injection of local anaesthetic is equivalent to an intravenous injection.

### Dural puncture

Puncture of the dura is more likely if:

(1) the dura extends to a lower level;
(2) the laminae of other sacral vertebrae are not fused so that the needle can be inadvertently inserted into the sacral canal at a higher segmental level;
(3) the caudal needle is inserted more than a few millimetres into the sacral canal.

Injection of a large dose of local anaesthetic into the subarachnoid space will produce a 'total spinal' block, characterized by sudden apnoea, unconsciousness, and dilated pupils. There is usually no haemodynamic disturbance in young children and babies, and the block resolves in 1–2 hours.

*Penetration of the sacrum*

The sacrum is cartilaginous and relatively soft. Penetration of the sacrum may damage pelvic viscera or blood vessels.

*Urinary retention*

In children who are well hydrated caudal bupivacaine 0.25 per cent does not delay micturition (Fisher *et al.* 1993).

*Paraesthesia and motor weakness*

Paraesthesia and motor weakness are more common with higher concentrations of local anaesthetic. Bupivacaine 0.125 per cent produces similar analgesia compared with bupivacaine 0.25 per cent but with significantly less motor weakness.

*Haematoma and infection*

Haematoma and abscess formation are very uncommon.

## Technique

The child lies in the left lateral position with the uppermost leg bent at right angles at the hip and knee joints and the lower leg bent at 120° (Fig. 12.10). The pelvis is rolled slightly away from the anaesthetist so that the lower part of the body is in a semi-prone position rotated slightly over the lower limb.

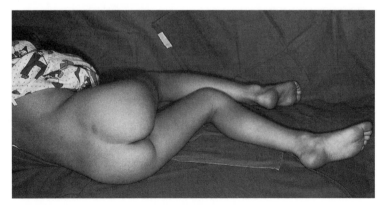

**Fig. 12.10**   Left lateral position for caudal extradural anaesthesia in children.

The sacral hiatus is located as a shallow depression at the apex of an equilateral triangle formed by the posterior superior iliac spines and in the mid-line at the end of a line running along the lateral border of the uppermost thigh (Fig. 12.11).

Some anaesthetists prefer a 21 g cutting needle without a stylet, and a small nick should be made in the skin before the caudal needle is inserted to reduce the risk of producing an implantation dermoid (Fig. 12.12).

*Insertion of the needle for caudal extradural anaesthesia in a child*

The caudal needle is inserted at the apex of the sacral hiatus, with its bevel facing anteriorly (Fig. 12.13). The sacrum in children is concave anteriorly and the caudal needle should be advanced in the sagittal plane at an angle of 45° to the skin, aiming in a cranial direction. A 'pop' is felt as the sacro-coccygeal membrane is

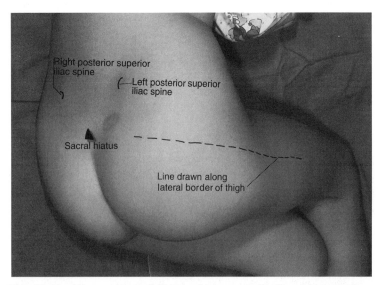

**Fig. 12.11**   The position of the sacral hiatus can be found by one of three methods: (a) at the apex of an equilateral triangle formed by the posterior superior iliac spines; (b) with the legs flexed at the hips the sacral hiatus lies in the mid-line at the end of a line drawn through the middle of the lateral thigh; (c) the sacral hiatus is can be palpated as a concave depression between the sacral cornua above the sacrococcygeal joint.

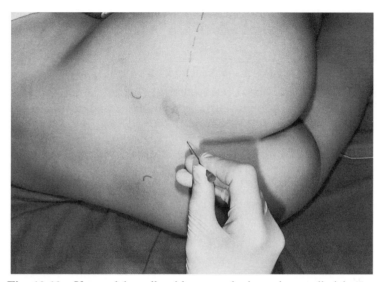

**Fig. 12.12**   If a caudal needle without a stylet is used, a small nick should be made in the skin before the caudal needle is inserted.

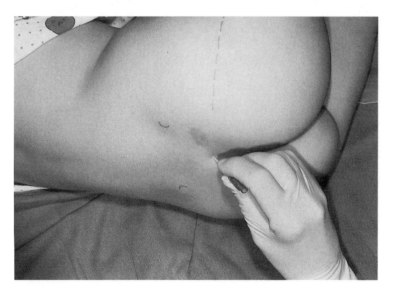

**Fig. 12.13**   Insertion of the needle for caudal extradural anaesthesia in a child. The needle is inserted at the apex of the sacral hiatus in a saggital plane at an angle of about 45° to the skin.

punctured. The needle should be advanced only about 3 mm into the sacral canal to reduce the risk of puncture of the venous plexus or dura.

*Insertion of the needle for caudal extradural anaesthesia in a baby*

The sacrum of a baby is relatively flat. The caudal needle should be inserted in the centre of the sacral hiatus and advanced in a sagittal plane at an angle of about 15° to the skin (Fig. 12.14).

If an intravenous cannula is used instead of a needle the cannula is advanced about 1 cm over the stylet once the sacro-coccygeal membrane is penetrated and the stylet then removed (Fig. 12.15). If the cannula cannot be advanced easily it is unlikely that it lies within the caudal extradural space and it should be re-inserted. 'Loss of resistance' to air or saline can be used to identify the extradural space. After gentle aspiration for cerebrospinal fluid and blood, local anaesthetic is injected slowly. There should be no resistance to injection. Gentle aspiration should be repeated throughout the injection: the pressure within extradural veins may be less than right atrial pressure when the child is in the lateral position and the vessel walls collapse easily.

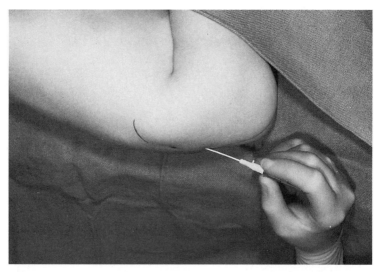

**Fig. 12.14**   Insertion of the needle for caudal extradural anaesthesia in a baby. The needle is inserted at the centre of the sacral hiatus in a saggital plane of about 15° to the skin.

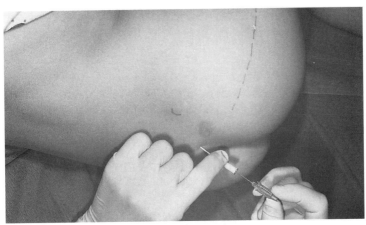

**Fig. 12.15** Using an intravenous cannula during caudal anaesthesia. Once the sacro-coccygeal membrane is penetrated, the cannula can be slid over the needle into the caudal space.

Catheters can be threaded through a cannula inserted through the sacral hiatus (Fig. 12.16). A 23 g catheter threads easily though a 20 g intravenous cannula. Increments of local anaesthetic can be given to extend the duration of anaesthesia.

Some anaesthetists prefer to make a second caudal injection at the end of surgery if the operation lasts longer than 2 hours. An

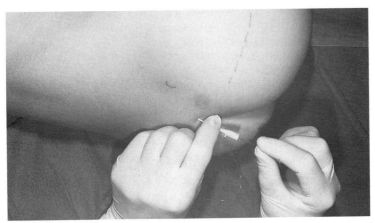

**Fig. 12.16** Extradural catheter can be threaded through a cannula inserted through the sacral hiatus.

equal volume of 0.125 per cent bupivacaine or half to two-thirds of the original volume of 0.25 per cent bupivacaine can be injected (maximum of 2.5 mg kg$^{-1}$ loading dose followed by 0.5 mg kg$^{-1}$ hour$^{-1}$).

## FURTHER READING

Arthur, D. S. and McNicol, L. R. (1986). Local anaesthetic techniques in paediatric surgery. *British Journal of Anaesthesia*, **58**, 760–78.

Yaster, M. and Maxwell, L. G. (1989). Pediatric regional anesthesia. *Anesthesiology*, **70**, 324–38.

## REFERENCES

Armitage, E. N. (1989). Regional anaesthesia. In *Textbook of paediatric anaesthetic practice*, (ed. E. Summer and D. Hatch), p. 217. Ballière Tindall, London.

Busoni, P. and Andreuccetti, T. (1986). The spread of caudal analgesia in children: a mathematical model. *Anaesthesia Intensive Care*, **14**, 140–4.

Dalens, B. and Hasnaoui, A. (1989). Caudal anesthesia in pediatric surgery: success rate and adverse effects in 750 consecutive patients. *Anesthesia Analgesia*, **68**, 83–9.

Eyres, R. L., Bishop, W., Oppenheim, R. C., and Brown, T. C. K. (1983). Plasma bupivacaine concentrations in children during caudal epidural analgesia. *Anaesthesia Intensive Care*, **11**, 20–2.

Fisher, Q. A. *et al.* (1993). Postoperative voiding interval and duration of analgesia following peripheral or caudal nerve blocks in children. *Anesthesia Analgesia*, **76**, 173–7.

Fortuna, A. (1989). Respiratory arrest after a caudal injection of bupivacaine. *Anaesthesia*, **44**, 1007.

Lee, E. and Collins G. (1990). Respiratory arrest after caudal bupivacaine. *Anaesthesia*, **45**, 63–4.

Lumb, A. B. and Carli, F. (1989). Respiratory arrest after a caudal injection of bupivacaine. *Anaesthesia*, **44**, 324–5.

Schulte-Steinberg, O. and Rahlfs, V. W. (1977). Spread of extradural analgesia following caudal injection in children. A statistical study. *British Journal of Anaesthesia*, **49**, 1027–33.

Takasaki, M., Dohi, S., Kawabata, Y., and Takahashi, T. (1977). Dosage of lidocaine for caudal anesthesia in infants and children. *Anesthesiology*, **47**, 527–9.

Warner, M. A., Kunkel, S. E., Offord, K. O., Atchison, S. R., and Dawson, B. (1987). The effects of age, epinephrine, and operative site on duration of caudal analgesia in pediatric patients. *Anesthesia Analgesia*, **66**, 995–8.

Wolf, A. R., Valley, R. D., Fear, D. W., Roy, W. L., and Lerman, J. (1988). Bupivacaine for caudal analgesia in infants and children: the optimal effective concentration. *Anesthesiology*, **69**, 102–6.

# CONTINUOUS EXTRADURAL ANAESTHESIA USING A CAUDAL APPROACH

## Introduction

Catheters can be threaded from the sacral hiatus to the lumbar or thoracic extradural spaces in babies and children up to 10 years of age. The tip of the catheter usually lies within one or two vertebral spaces of the desired segmental level.

## Indications

### Thoracic or abdominal operations in babies younger than 6 months

The technique of continuous extradural analgesia using a caudal approach is particularly useful in young babies because:

(1)  a conventional approach to the lumbar or thoracic extradural spaces is difficult and there is probably a higher risk of dural puncture or damage to the spinal cord;
(2)  using a single injection of local anaesthetic into the caudal extradural space to block thoracic dermatomes is not recommended because:
    (a)  large volumes of local anaesthetic are needed;
    (b)  increments of local anaesthetic cannot be injected to prolong the duration of block;
    (c)  the duration of analgesia is short in the upper segments.

A lumbar approach to the extradural space is preferred in babies older than 6 months because this technique avoids the potential risk of contamination of the catheter site with faeces.

### Lengthy surgery within the lower lumbar or sacral dermatomes

The block produced by a single caudal or intrathecal injection of local anaesthetic may not last long enough for complex perineal or penile surgery. Increments of local anaesthetic can be injected through a catheter to prolong the duration of block.

## Contraindications

(1)  Local infection;
(2)  septicaemia;

(3)  coagulopathy;
(4)  hydrocephalus;
(5)  meningomyelocoele;
(6)  local neurological disease;
(7)  uncorrected hypovolaemia;
(8)  major malformations of the sacrum.

## Equipment

Extradural catheters are threaded easily from the sacral hiatus through intravenous cannulae or brachial plexus catheter introducers. These techniques have several advantages compared with using Tuohy needles:

(1)  the sacrum in babies is relatively flat and it is easier to enter the sacral canal with a needle advanced at 10–15° to the skin. A cannula with an end-hole is probably more likely than a Tuohy needle to guide the catheter cranially;
(2)  the catheter can be removed and re-threaded without risk of shearing;
(3)  in babies who are awake the cannula can be advanced 1–1.5 cm into the extradural space and is unlikely to become dislodged if the baby moves.

Examples of suitable equipment include:

(1)  20 g intravenous cannula without 'wings' (e.g. Abbocath-T®, Abbot Laboratories) and a 23 g extradural catheter;
(2)  18 g intravenous cannula and a 20 g extradural catheter;
(3)  20 g brachial plexus catheter kit with an 18 g introducing cannula (e.g. Contiplex®, B. Braun Med Ltd).

## Drugs

Bupivacaine 0.25 per cent is commonly used for extradural anaesthesia in babies and children. The initial dose and subsequent rates of infusion are discussed on pp. 191–3.

## Complications

Many of the general complications of lumbar epidural and caudal block apply also to the technique of continuous extradural anaesthesia using a caudal approach (see pp. 194–6 and 208–9). The specific complications of the technique of continuous extradural anaesthesia using a caudal approach are:

*Intravenous or subarachnoid placement of the catheter*

Unrecognized intravenous or subarachnoid placement of the catheter can result in seizures, ventricular fibrillation, or ventilatory arrest when local anaesthetic is injected. Some authors use X-ray contrast to confirm the position of the catheter tip or a test dose of local anaesthetic containing 1 : 200 000 adrenaline (0.1 ml kg$^{-1}$) to exclude intravascular injection. However, in children anaesthetized with halothane a test dose may be unreliable unless atropine has been given first (see p. 193). A test dose is probably even more unreliable in awake babies.

To reduce the risk of toxicity, the following precautions should be taken when injecting local anaesthetic:

(1)  aspirate the catheter gently before injecting local anaesthetic and repeatedly during the injection;

(2)  inject the local anaethetic slowly (over 5–10 minutes) to reduce the peak concentration. The risk of toxic side-effects correlates with the peak concentration, and the peak concentration for a given dose of local anaesthetic depends on the rate of injection.

The incidence of intravascular or subarachnoid placement of the catheter is not known. Bösenberg and colleagues (1992) sited catheters through 18 g cannulae and reported no clinical evidence of catheter misplacements among 160 babies (including 85 neonates). However, van Niekerk and colleagues (1990) used Tuohy needles and found on epidurography an incidence of unrecognized subarachnoid or intravascular placement of 2 of 20 catheters. Van Niekerk's technique differed from that of other authors as follows:

(1)  the catheters were sited with the babies in a 20° head-down tilt. In this position the extradural veins may collapse and blood may not be drawn along the lumen when the catheter is aspirated;

(2)  the sacral canal was cannulated with a Tuohy needle rather than an end-holed cannula;

(3)  the babies were very small (weight 520–2750 g).

*Contamination of catheter site with faecal bacteria*

Contamination of catheter site with faecal bacteria is a potential risk.

## Difficulties

*Inability to advance the catheter to the appropriate segmental level*
Inability to thread the catheter is usually caused by:

(1)  the introducing cannula lying outside the sacral canal;
(2)  resistance between the catheter and cannula;
(3)  the tip of the catheter impinging against a nerve root—if the catheter is forcibly advanced against a resistance it may damage nerve roots, double back, or form a loop.

An obstruction may be overcome by:

(1)  removing the catheter and injecting sterile 0.9 per cent sodium chloride through the cannula to act as a lubricant,
(2)  pulling the catheter back slightly and gently flexing, extending, or stretching the child's back within the normal range of movement and then re-advancing the catheter.

If the catheter cannot be threaded to the appropriate segmental level it can be pulled back slightly and left in place. A larger volume of local anaesthetic can then be injected to obtain an adequate height of block.

### Kinking of the catheter

Kinking of the catheter after placement is more common with small-bore catheters and can prevent injection of local anaesthetic.

### Technique

An assistant holds the baby in the left lateral position with the hips flexed but the head reasonably extended to prevent oxygen desaturation in awake babies, or movement of the tracheal tube in anaesthetized babies (Fig. 12.17). The skin of the lower back, natal cleft, and buttocks are thoroughly cleaned with an alcoholic antiseptic solution and the area draped with sterile towels. The distance from the sacral hiatus to the desired level for the tip of the catheter is measured with the extradural catheter.

In awake babies the skin overlying the sacral hiatus is infiltrated with 1 per cent lignocaine using a 27 g needle. A 20 g intravenous cannula is advanced through the sacral hiatus in a sagittal plane at

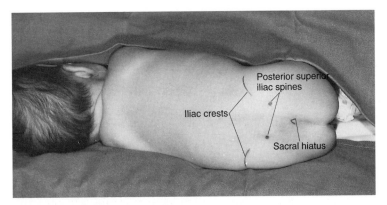

**Fig. 12.17** Position and landmarks for continuous caudal extradural analgesia in babies.

an angle of 10–15° to the skin (Fig. 12.18). A 'pop' is felt as the shoulders of the cannula pass through the sacro-coccygeal membrane. The sacro-coccygeal membrane is approximately 5 mm from the skin in neonates and 5–10 mm in older children.

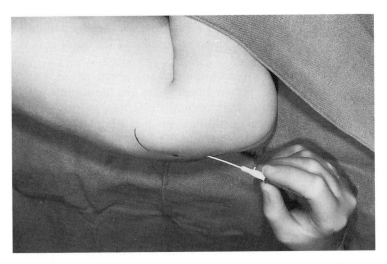

**Fig. 12.18** An intravenous cannula inserted through the sacral hiatus can be used to site extradural catheters. The cannula should be advanced through the hiatus at an angle of about 15° to the skin.

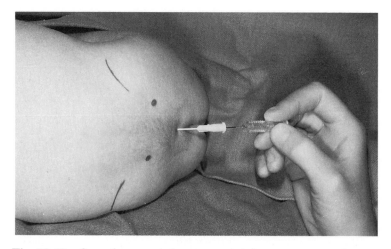

**Fig. 12.19** Once the cannula has penetrated the sacro-coccygeal membrane it should be advanced a further 3 mm and then flattened against the skin. The cannula is then slid 1–1.5 cm over the needle into the caudal space.

The needle is advanced a further 3 mm and then flattened against the skin. The cannula is advanced 1–1.5 cm over the needle (Fig. 12.19). It should advance easily if it lies within the sacral canal. The needle is then removed and the cannula gently aspirated with a syringe.

If neither blood nor cerebrospinal fluid appears in the syringe, an extradural catheter is then threaded through the cannula so that its tip lies a few centimetres beyond the desired segmental level (Fig. 12.20). To prevent nerve damage or looping of the catheter, the catheter should NEVER be forced against an obstruction. The cannula is carefully removed and the catheter pulled back so that the desired length lies within the extradural space. The open end of the catheter is held for 1–2 minutes below the level of the baby and the lumen examined for cerebrospinal fluid and blood. The catheter is then gently aspirated with a syringe.

The catheter is secured in a loop with a waterproof, transparent dressing so that the site of entry can be examined easily and is isolated from potential faecal contaminants (Fig. 12.21). Local anaesthetic is slowly injected through a bacterial filter into the extradural space. An infusion or incremental doses of local anaesthetic can then be given.

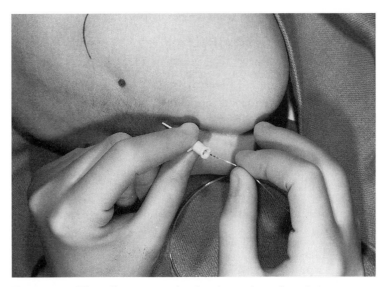

**Fig. 12.20**   Threading an extradural catheter through an intravenous cannula inserted through the sacral hiatus.

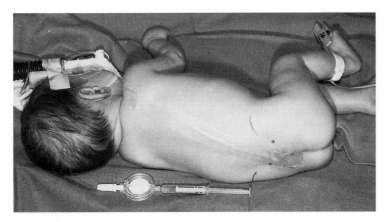

**Fig. 12.21**   A caudal extradural catheter secured in a loop with a water proof, transparent dressing. Local anaesthetic is injected through a 0.22 μm filter.

# REFERENCES

Bösenberg, A. T., Bland, B. A. R., Schulte-Steinberg, O., and Downing, J. W. (1988). Thoracic epidural anesthesia via caudal route in infants. *Anesthesiology*, **69**, 265–9.

Bösenberg, A. T., Hadley, G. P., and Wiersma, R. (1992). Oesophageal atresia: caudo-thoracic epidural anaesthesia reduces the need for post-operative ventilatory support. *Pediatric Surgery International*, 7, 289–91.

Desparmet, J., Mateo, J., Ecoffey, C., and Mazoit, X. (1990). Efficacy of an epidural test dose in children anesthetised with halothane. *Anesthesiology*, **72**, 249–51.

Gunter, J. B. and Eng, C. (1992). Thoracic epidural anesthesia via the caudal approach in children. *Anesthesiology*, **76**, 935–8.

Peutrell, J. M. and Hughes, D. G. (1993). Epidural anaesthesia through caudal catheters in awake ex-premature babies. *Anaesthesia*, **47**, 128–31.

Rasch, D. K., Webster, D. E., Pollard, T. G., and Gurkowski, M. A. (1990). Lumbar and thoracic epidural analgesia via the caudal approach for postoperative pain relief in infants and children. *Canadian Journal of Anaesthesia*, **37**, 359–62.

Van Niekerk, J., Bax-Vermeire, B. M. J., Geurts, J. W. M., and Kramer, P. P. G. (1990). Epidurography in premature infants. *Anaesthesia*, **45**, 722–5.

# OTHER EXTRADURAL AND INTRATHECAL DRUGS

## Opioids

Opioids act on specific receptors within the substantia gelatinosa of the dorsal horn of the spinal cord (spinal receptors) and in the brain (supra-spinal receptors). The action of opioids on spinal receptors produces segmental analgesia without blocking autonomic, motor, or other sensory functions. Profound analgesia occurs with low plasma concentrations compared with those normally associated with systemic analgesia. This supports the view that the main site of action of extradural and intrathecal opioids is at spinal receptors. Opioids and local anaesthetics have a synergistic action.

Morphine is the most common drug injected into the subarachnoid or extradural space in children. The duration of analgesia is considerably longer than after intravenous or intramuscular morphine.

*Extradural*

Extradural opioids have a biphasic action: the initial effect is due to systemic absorption and the sustained effect is caused by specific binding to spinal receptors.

Preservative-free morphine up to 100 $\mu$g kg$^{-1}$ can be injected into the caudal extradural space to provide analgesia after operations below the diaphragm. The duration of analgesia is usually longer than 10 hours and can exceed 24 hours. Clinically satisfactory analgesia can be obtained at the lower dose with potentially less risk of serious side-effects. Caudal morphine 70 and 75 $\mu$g kg$^{-1}$ (usually combined with intraoperative opioids) has been given to obtain prolonged analgesia after thoracotomy. This technique probably relies upon the cephalad spread of morphine within the cerebrospinal fluid.

Morphine can be injected through extradural catheters positioned at lumbar or thoracic level to provide analgesia after operations on the thorax, abdomen, or legs. An injection of 25–50 $\mu$g kg$^{-1}$ produces analgesia usually lasting more than 15 hours and this dose can be repeated if necessary.

Diamorphine can be injected into the extradural space to provide analgesia. An initial injection of 25 $\mu$g kg$^{-1}$ can be given at the thoracic level and 50 $\mu$g kg$^{-1}$ at the lumbar level. This can be followed by a postoperative infusion of 5–25 $\mu$g kg$^{-1}$ h$^{-1}$ in combination with local anaesthetic (equivalent to 3 mg of diamorphine in 60 ml local anaesthetic infused at a rate of 0.1–0.5 ml kg$^{-1}$ h$^{-1}$).

*Intrathecal morphine*

Preservative-free morphine 20–30 $\mu$g kg$^{-1}$ can be injected into the lumbar subarachnoid space to provide prolonged analgesia after cardiac surgery, cranio-facial reconstruction, laparotomy, or correction of subglottic stenosis. The technique relies upon the spread of morphine within the cerebrospinal fluid to higher segmental levels, and there is a potential risk of ventilatory depression. The duration of analgesia is longer than 12 hours in most children.

## Complications and side-effects

*Ventilatory depression*

The risk of ventilatory depression after spinal opioids in children is not known. The incidence associated with repeated injections of extradural morphine in adults is about 0.2 per cent but is uncommon more than 6 hours after injection. The incidence is probably greater:

(1)  in babies
(2)  if additional opioids are given by other routes; and
(3)  if opioids are delivered at higher segmental levels (i.e. through extradural catheters).

Ventilatory depression can occur in the absence of other risk factors: it has been reported in a 2.5-year-old boy who had caudal morphine 100 $\mu$g kg$^{-1}$ and who was not given opioids by other route.

The ventilatory effects of extradural opioids are biphasic: early depression is due to systemic absorption and late depression is caused by cephalad spread within the cerebrospinal fluid. Late-onset ventilatory depression after extradural morphine in children occurs at about $3\frac{1}{2}$ hours and can be sudden. This is much quicker than in adults and may be explained by more rapid cephalad spread of morphine. More lipid-soluble opioids (e.g. diamorphine) can also depress breathing.

Ventilatory depression can be treated with intravenous naloxone 2–20 $\mu$g kg$^{-1}$ followed by an infusion of 2–10 $\mu$g kg$^{-1}$ h$^{-1}$.

### Pruritus

Pruritus occurs in about 20–30 per cent of children given extradural morphine. It often affects the face and can be very distressing. It can be treated with intravenous naloxone 1–2 $\mu$g kg$^{-1}$ followed by an infusion of 1–2 $\mu$g kg$^{-1}$ h$^{-1}$, without impairing the quality of analgesia.

### Urinary retention

The incidence of urinary retention after caudal morphine is about 30 per cent but this is not significantly different compared with caudal bupivacaine or intravenous morphine. The incidence may be higher when morphine is injected at a higher segmental level.

Urinary retention associated with opioids can be treated with an intravenous infusion of naloxone 2–5 $\mu$g kg$^{-1}$ h$^{-1}$.

### Nausea and vomiting

The incidence of nausea and vomiting in children given a single injection of caudal morphine is not significantly different from that in children given intravenous morphine or caudal bupivacaine. A higher rate of nausea and vomiting is associated with extradural morphine given at a higher segmental level.

Nausea and vomiting may be reduced by oral premedication with a mixture of trimeprazine 3 mg kg$^{-1}$ and droperidol 0.15 mg kg$^{-1}$ or can be treated with intravenous naloxone 2–5 $\mu$g kg$^{-1}$ h$^{-1}$ with only a slight reduction in the duration of analgesia.

## FURTHER READING

McIlvaine, W. B. (1990). Spinal opioids for the pediatric patient. *Journal of Pain and Symptom Management*, 5, 183–90.

## REFERENCES

Dalens, B. and Chrysostome, Y. (1991). Intervertebral epidural anaesthesia in paediatric surgery: success rate and adverse effects in 650 consecutive procedures. *Paediatric Anaesthesia*, 1, 107–17.

Dalens, B., Tanguy, A., and Haberer, J.-P. (1986). Lumbar epidural anesthesia for operative and postoperative pain relief in infants and young children. *Anesthesia Analgesia*, 65, 1069–73.

Irving, G. A., Butt, A. D., and Van der Veen, B. (1993). A comparison of caudal morphine given pre- or post-surgery for postoperative analgesia in children. *Paediatric Anaesthesia*, 3, 217–21.

Jensen, B. H. (1981). Caudal block for post-operative pain relief in children after genital operations. A comparison between bupivacaine and morphine. *Acta Anaesthesiologica Scandinavica*, 25, 373–5.

Jones, S. E. F., Beasley, J. M., MacFarlane, D. W. R., Davis, J. M., and Hall-Davies, G. (1984). Intrathecal morphine for postoperative pain relief in children. *British Journal of Anaesthesia*, 56, 137–40.

Krane, E. J. (1988). Delayed respiratory depression in a child after caudal epidural morphine. *Anesthesia Analgesia*, 67, 79–82.

Krane, E. J., Jacobson, L. E., Lynn, A. M., Parrot, C., and Tyler, D. C. (1987). Caudal morphine for postoperative analgesia in children: a comparison with caudal bupivacaine and intravenous morphine. *Anesthesia Analgesia*, 66, 647–53.

Krane, E. J., Tyler, D. C., and Jacobson, L. E. (1989). The dose response of caudal morphine in children. *Anesthesiology*, 71, 48–52.

Krechel, S. W. and Helikson, M. A. (1993). Intrathecal morphine for pain control in term infants for oesophageal atresia/tracheo-oesophageal fistula repair. *Paediatric Anaesthesia*, 3, 243–7.

Rasch, D. K., Webster, D. E., Pollard, T. G., and Gurkowski, M. A. (1990). Lumbar and thoracic epidural analgesia via the caudal approach for postoperative pain relief in infants and children. *Canadian Journal of Anaesthesia*, **37**, 359–62.

Ready, L. B., Loper, K. A., Nessly, M., and Wild, L. (1991). Postoperative epidural morphine, is it safe on surgical wards? *Anesthesiology*, **75**, 452–6.

Rose, J. B., Francis, M. C., and Kettrick, R. G. (1993). Continuous naloxone infusion in paediatric patients with pruritus associated with epidural morphine. *Paediatric Anaesthesia*, **3**, 255–8.

Rosen, K. R. and Rosen, D. A. (1989). Caudal epidural morphine for control of pain following open heart surgery in children. *Anesthesiology*, **70**, 418–21.

Tobias, J. D., Deshpande, J. K., Wetzel, R. C., Facker, J., Maxwell, L. G., and Solca, M. (1990). Postoperative analgesia. Use of intrathecal morphine in children. *Clinical Pediatrics*, **29**, 44–8.

Valley, R. D. and Bailey, A. G. (1991). Caudal morphine for postoperative analgesia in infants and children: a report of 138 cases. *Anesthesia Analgesia*, **72**, 120–4.

Wilson, P. T. J. and Lloyd-Thomas, A. R. (1993). An audit of extradural infusion analgesia in children using bupivacaine and diamorphine. *Anaesthesia*, **48**, 718–23.

Wolf, A. R., Hughes, D., Hobbs, A. J., and Prys-Roberts, C. (1991). Combined morphine-bupivacaine caudals for reconstructive penile surgery in children: systemic absorption of morphine and postoperative analgesia. *Anaesthesia Intensive Care*, **19**, 17–21.

## Ketamine

Ketamine is an $N$-methyl-D-aspartate receptor antagonist that modulates nociception in the spinal cord. Ketamine 0.5 mg kg$^{-1}$ injected into the caudal extradural space is not associated with motor weakness, urinary retention, or behavioural changes, and produces analgesia comparable to bupivacaine 0.25 per cent. Ketamine may cause neurotoxicity, which would limit the use of this technique.

## REFERENCES

Malinovsky, J. M. *et al.* (1991). Ketamine and midazolam neurotoxicity in the rabbit. *Anesthesiology*, **75**, 91–7.

Naguib, M., Sharif, A. M. Y., Seraj, M., El Gammal, M., and Dawlatly, A. A. (1991). Ketamine for caudal analgesia in children: comparison with caudal bupivacaine. *British Journal of Anaesthesia*, **67**, 559–64.

## Clonidine

Clonidine is an $\alpha_2$ adrenergic agonist with peripheral and central nervous system effects. Clonidine acts in the central nervous system on inhibitory receptors in the substantia gelatinosa of the spinal cord and supra-spinal receptors in the medulla to modulate pain transmission. When injected into the subarachnoid or extradural space it produces analgesia without blocking motor or proprioceptive pathways. It is not associated with nausea, vomiting, pruritus or ventilatory depression but can produce hypotension and sedation in adults. Subarachnoid and extradural clonidine potentiates the analgesic effects of local anaesthetics and opioids but is not usually adequate for postoperative analgesia when given alone.

Caudal clonidine has been evaluated in children in only two studies: 1–2 $\mu$g kg$^{-1}$ significantly prolonged the duration of caudal bupivacaine without increasing unpleasant side-effects. Clonidine probably increases postoperative sedation in children.

Further research is needed to assess the safety and use of this technique in children.

## REFERENCES

Jamali, S., Monin, S., Begon, C., Dubousset, A.-M., and Ecoffey, C. (1994) Clonidine in pediatric caudal anesthesia. *Anesthesia Analgesia*, **78**, 663–6.

Lee, J. J. and Rubin, A. P. (1994). Comparison of a bupivacaine–clonidine mixture with plain bupivacaine for caudal analgesia in children. *British Journal of Anaesthesia*, **72**, 258–62.

# POSTOPERATIVE MANAGEMENT OF CHILDREN GIVEN CONTINUOUS EXTRADURAL ANALGESIA OR SPINAL OPIOIDS

## *Quality of analgesia*

Infusions or intermittent injections of local anaesthetics (alone or combined with opioids) can be given through extradural catheters to provide analgesia after surgery. Continuous lumbar extradural infusions of bupivacaine produce analgesia comparable to an intravenous morphine infusion but with less sedation and higher oxygen saturations.

### Rates of infusion of local anaesthetic in children and babies older than 1 month

A loading dose of $0.5-1.0$ ml kg$^{-1}$ of bupivacaine 0.25 per cent with a subsequent infusion rate of $0.1-0.2$ ml kg$^{-1}$ h$^{-1}$ ($= 0.25-0.50$ mg kg$^{-1}$) usually provides good analgesia. There is no evidence that children are more resistant to the toxic effects of local anaesthetic than adults and a maximum rate of infusion of $0.5$ mg kg$^{-1}$ h$^{-1}$ should not be exceeded.

### Rates of infusion of local anaesthetic in babies younger than 4 weeks

Young babies are potentially at greater risk of toxic side–effects because they have lower concentrations of binding proteins (principally alpha$_1$ acid glycoprotein) and a higher free fraction of local anaesthetic. The maximum recommended loading dose of bupivacaine in neonates is $2.5$ mg kg$^{-1}$ and the subsequent rate of infusion should be less than $0.2$ mg kg$^{-1}$ h$^{-1}$.

### Course of action if analgesia is inadequate

If the analgesia is inadequate despite the maximum rate of infusion, the following can be tried:

(1) continuing with the extradural infusion of local anaesthetic and injecting opioids either intravenously or through the catheter (see pp. 222–6);
(2) giving non-steroidal analgesics in addition to extradural analgesia;
(3) abandoning the extradural infusion of local anaesthetic in favour of non-steroidal analgesic drugs or opioids given by another route.

### Postoperative monitoring and nursing care

Children with continuous infusions of epidural local anaesthetics can be nursed on surgical wards where children are cared for after major surgical operations if the following precautions are taken:

(1) nurses must be trained to recognize the complications associated with extradural analgesia and in the immediate resuscitation of children;

(2) medical staff trained in resusitation of children must be available at all times;

(3) each bed space should be equipped with oxygen and suction;

(4) the ward must have adequate equipment and drugs to treat cardiorespiratory arrest, convulsions, and hypotension;

(5) naloxone should be available if spinal opioids have been given;

(6) the child should be assessed at least once a day by a pain nurse or an anaesthetist and the ward staff should have clear instructions on whom to call if there is a problem.

Postoperative monitoring should include continuous pulse oximetry and measurements of:

(1) blood pressure;
(2) heart rate;
(3) ventilatory rate;
(4) quality of pain control;
(5) sedation.

These measurements should be made hourly for 12 hours, 2 hourly for the next 12 hours, and 4 hourly thereafter. The postoperative observation chart and analgesia guidelines used with extradural infusions at the Royal Hospital for Sick Children, Bristol, are shown in Fig. 12.22.

If infusions of extradural opioids are given, the level of sedation must be regularly assessed and some authors recommend using an apnoea monitor. Opioids must not be given by another route without consultation with an anaesthetist.

Spinal opioids should be used with great care in babies younger than 12 months because of the greater risk of ventilatory depression. These babies should be nursed on a high dependency or intensive care unit for the duration of a continuous infusion of spinal opioid or for 12–24 hours after a single injection. Monitoring should include continuous oximetry and an apnoea alarm.

Absence of sedation despite an adequate sensory block may make young children difficult to nurse, particularly with infusions containing bupivacaine only. Agitation is the usual cause of the failure of the technique postoperatively. Morphine has analgesic

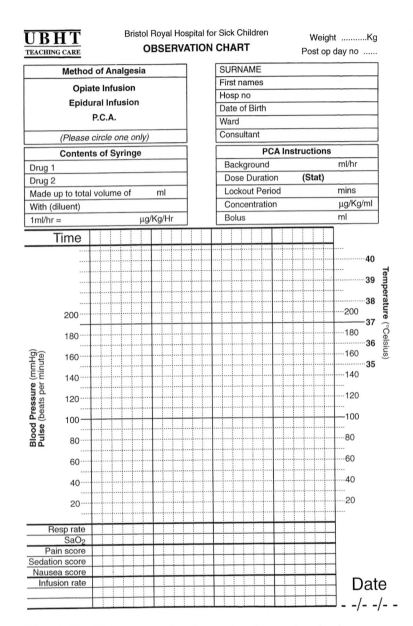

**Fig. 12.22** The postoperative observation chart and analgesia guidelines used with extradural infusions at the Royal Hospital for Sick Children, Bristol.

## Postoperative Analgesia Guidelines

**Monitoring**  Hourly for the first 12 hours,
2 hourly until 24 hours,
then 4 hourly.

**Pain score**  0 = Nil
1 = Mild
2 = Moderate
3 = Severe

**Sedation score**  0 = Awake and alert
1 = Occasionally drowsy, easy to arouse
2 = Drowsy most of the time, easy to arouse
3 = Somnolent, difficult to arouse

**Nausea score**  0 = None
1 = Nausea
2 = Vomiting

# Management

> **Call the on call Anaesthetist if: -**
>
> **1) Respiratory rate less than   10 / 15 / 20**
>
> **2) Pain score = 3**
>
> **3) Sedation score = 3**

Changes in prescriptions can only be made by a member of the Anaesthetic staff.

The infusion rate can be adjusted in response to the patient's pain by a member of the nursing staff.

The analgesic regimen should be continued for 12 - 72 hours according to the instructions of the Anaesthetic team. After this time, if the patient is comfortable and there are no complications, then the epidural / iv infusion / PCA may be discontinued.

Alternative analgesia should be available before infusion is withdrawn.

and sedative properties. Intravenous injections of 50–100 $\mu$g kg$^{-1}$ can be useful in agitated children if intrathecal or extradural opioids have not been given.

### Serious complications

Migration of catheters, or excessively high blocks can occur postoperatively. Accumulation of local anaesthetic with the risk of systemic toxicity can occur occasionally in normal children. The maximum rates of infusion should be reduced in children with reduced clearance (e.g. hepatic resection), or increased risk of convulsions (e.g. epilepsy, pyrexia in children with febrile convulsions).

Serious complications associated with spinal opioids are discussed on pp. 223–4.

### Technical problems

Technical problems account for the loss of up to 17 per cent of extradural infusions in children after surgery, and include:

(1) malplaced catheters or unilateral or patchy blocks that do not become apparent until after operation;
(2) leakage from the puncture site occurs in about 7 per cent; this can usually be compensated for by a bolus injection and increasing the infusion rate;
(3) occluded catheters (usually due to kinking of the catheter);
(4) catheter-connector disconnections, with a risk of contamination of the catheter.

Many of these problems are more common with catheters of small bore.

## REFERENCES

Agarwal, R., Gutlove, D. P., and Lockhart, C. H. (1992). Seizures occurring in pediatric patients receiving continuous infusion of bupivacaine. *Anesthesia Analgesia*, **75**, 284–6.

Desparmet, J., Meistelman, C., Barre, J., and Saint-Maurice, C. (1987). Continuous epidural infusion of bupivacaine for postoperative pain relief in children. *Anesthesiology*, **67**, 108–10.

Mazoit, J. X., Denson, D. D., and Samii, K. (1988). Pharmacokinetics of bupivacaine following caudal anesthesia in infants. *Anesthesiology*, **68**, 387–91.

Wilson, P. T. J. and Lloyd-Thomas, A. R. (1993). An audit of extradural infusion analgesia in children using bupivacaine and diamorphine. *Anaesthesia*, **48**, 718–23.

Wolf, A. R. and Hughes, D. (1993). Pain relief for infants undergoing abdominal surgery: comparison of infusions of I. V. morphine and extradural bupivacaine. *British Journal of Anaesthesia*, **70**, 10–16.

Wolf, A. R. *et al.* (1993). Effect of extradural analgesia on stress responses to abdominal surgery in infants. *British Journal of Anaesthesia*, **70**, 654–60.

# 13

# *Subarachnoid anaesthesia in children*

## J. M. PEUTRELL

## INTRODUCTION

Subarachnoid anaesthesia has been used in children since the early part of this century but is no longer popular because:

(1) the duration of analgesia produced by a single injection of local anaesthetic is short and insufficient for postoperative pain control;

(2) general anaesthesia is usually used in children.

Subarachnoid block is indicated:

(1) to provide prolonged analgesia using intrathecal opioids in older children having major surgery (see p. 223)

(2) in awake ex-premature babies using local anaesthetic solutions in an attempt to reduce the risk of postoperative apnoea (see pp. 236–48).

### *Anatomy*

In full-term babies, the spinal cord extends to L3 and the dura to S3 or S4. At about 12 months of age the terminations of the spinal cord and dura reach the adult positions of L1 or L2, and S2, respectively. A lumbar puncture can be made at the L2–L3, L3–L4, or L4–L5 interspaces in children and L3–L4, L4–L5, L5–S1, or S1–S2 interspaces in babies. The intercristal line usually crosses L5 in young children and L5–S1 in babies.

The technique of lumbar puncture in children is similar to that used in adults. Post-lumbar-puncture headache is uncommon but the risk of headache can be reduced in older children by using atraumatic needles (e.g. Whitacre or Sprotte of small diameter. Intrathecal opioids are discussed on pp. 222–3.

## REFERENCES

Ghia, J. N., Spielman, F. J., and Stieber, S. F. (1984). The diagnosis and successful treatment of post-lumbar puncture headache in a paediatric patient. *Regional Anesthesia*, **9**, 102–5.

Gray, H. T. (1909). A study of spinal anaesthesia in children and infants. From a series of 200 cases. *Lancet*, **ii**, 913–17.

Jones, S. E. F., Beasley, J. M., MacFarlane, D. W. R., Davis, J. M., and Hall-Davies, G. (1984). Intrathecal morphine for postoperative pain relief in children. *British Journal of Anaesthesia*, **56**, 137–40.

Tobias, J. D., Deshpande, J. K., Wetzel, R. C., Facker J., Maxwell, L. G., and Solca, M. (1990). Postoperative analgesia. Use of intrathecal morphine in children. *Clinical Paediatrics*, **29**, 44–8.

# 14

# *Regional anaesthesia in awake babies*

## J. M. PEUTRELL

## INTRODUCTION

Babies born before 37 weeks' gestation are at risk of postoperative apnoea, and regional anaesthetic techniques have been recommended to reduce this risk.

Apnoea is usually defined as either:

(1) the cessation of breathing for 15 seconds or longer; or
(2) the cessation of breathing for a shorter period if associated with bradycardia or cyanosis.

Postoperative apnoea in ex-premature babies has several clinical characteristics:

(1) the incidence is inversely related to the post-conceptional age of the baby at the time of surgery and not the gestational age at birth;
(2) the risk of postoperative apnoea persists up to 55 weeks' post-conceptional age;
(3) the first apnoea occurs within 12 hours of surgery, usually within the first 2 hours;
(4) if a baby has one episode of apnoea, the risk of further episodes persists for longer in younger babies;
(5) the preoperative breathing pattern will not predict babies at risk;
(6) postoperative apnoea can occur in babies with no history of idiopathic apnoea of prematurity;
(7) no association has yet been shown between the incidence of postoperative apnoea and the drugs used for general

anaesthesia (except for ketamine), or the preoperative condition of the baby.

Postoperative apnoea affects about a quarter of ex-premature babies younger than 44 weeks, post-conception, but in the absence of neurological disease is uncommon in babies older than 48 weeks' post-conception. The incidence after minor surgery is probably reduced by regional anaesthetic techniques without sedation, compared with general anaesthesia, but apnoea can still occur. Caudal extradural and subarachnoid blocks have been used to provide anaesthesia in babies having lower abdominal or perineal surgery (e.g. inguinal herniotomy or circumcision).

## GENERAL ASPECTS OF SUBARACHNOID AND CAUDAL EXTRADURAL ANAESTHESIA IN AWAKE BABIES

### *Preoperative preparation*

Babies are fed 4 hours, and given clear fluids 2 hours, before surgery so that they are not irritable and unsettled during the operation because of hunger. Sedation probably increases the incidence of postoperative apnoea and sedative premedication should not be prescribed routinely.

### *Monitoring*

The electrocardiograph should be monitored before starting the regional technique. Blood pressure measurements and oxygen saturation monitoring are often unreliable before a block has developed, because of movement. A blood pressure cuff can be applied to the leg and a oximetry probe to the foot after injecting the local anaesthetic. Inflation of the cuff will not disturb the baby once the sensory block has developed.

### *Induction of anaesthesia*

An intravenous cannula should be inserted before a caudal block because of the risks of local anaesthetic toxicity or a 'total spinal'. This may not be necessary with a subarachnoid block because of the smaller doses of local anaesthetic used, and a cannula can be sited in the leg once the block is effective. Hypotension is not usually a feature of either caudal extradural or subarachnoid block in babies.

The babies should be held firmly by a well-trained assistant. Lumbar puncture can be made with the babies in the sitting or lateral positions (see Figs 14.1 and 14.2) and during caudal block they can be held over the assistant's shoulder or in the lateral position (see Figs 14.5 and 14.6). The babies' hips are flexed but the head should be slightly extended to prevent oxygen desaturation.

### *Intraoperative management*

Babies often sleep during surgery, possibly because of the sensory de-afferentation. Awake babies can be comforted with a 'dummy'.

The motor block associated with a caudal extradural block is often incomplete and the upper thighs should be gently restrained with padding and tape to prevent movement of the legs interfering with surgery.

Intravenous fluids (e.g. glucose 5 per cent and NaCl 0.225 per cent) should be infused at a rate according to weight and duration of fast.

Caudal extradural or subarachnoid blocks alone provide satisfactory anaesthesia in about 80–90 per cent of babies. Other local anaesthetic blocks (e.g. iliac crest block, infiltration of the spermatic cord or peritoneum) or sedation (inhalational or intravenous) are given in up to 10 per cent of babies because the duration or height of the central block is inadequate. Most problems occur during deep dissection of the hernial sac or traction on the peritoneum or spermatic cord. General anaesthesia is used in up to 10 per cent, either because the caudal or subarachnoid spaces cannot be found or because the subsequent block is inadequate.

### *Postoperative monitoring*

The risk of postoperative apnoea after regional anaesthesia without sedation in awake ex-premature babies is probably reduced but not eliminated. Sedatives or general anaesthesia may increase the risk. Babies should be monitored with pulse oximetry and apnoea alarms until 12 hours have elapsed without apnoea. The monitors should be set to alarm if:

(1) breathing ceases for longer than 15 seconds; or
(2) the pulse rate falls below 100 beats minute$^{-1}$; or
(3) the oxygen saturation is below 90 per cent.

## Postoperative analgesia

Paracetamol 15 mg kg$^{-1}$ (orally or rectally) should be given every 6 hours, starting immediately after surgery.

## FURTHER READING

Welborn, L. G. (1992). Post-operative apnoea in the former preterm infant: a review. *Paediatric Anaesthesia*, **2**, 37–44.
Gregory, G. A. and Steward, D. J. (1983). Life-threatening perioperative apnea in the ex-'premie'. Anesthesiology, **59**, 495–8.

## REFERENCES

Cox, R. G. and Goresky, G. V. (1990). Life-threatening apnea following spinal anesthesia in former premature infants. *Anesthesiology*, **73**, 345–7.
Gleason, C. A., Martin, R. J., Anderson, J.V., Carlo, W.A., Sanniti, K. J., and Fanaroff, A. A. (1983). Optimal position for a spinal tap in preterm infants. *Pediatrics*, **71**, 31–5.
Kurth, C. D., Spitzer, A. R., Broennle, A. M., and Downes, J. J. (1987). Postoperative apnea in preterm babies. *Anesthesiology*, **66**, 483–8.
Malviya, S., Swartz, J., and Lerman, J. (1993). Are all preterm infants younger than 60 weeks postconceptual age at risk for postanesthetic apnea? *Anesthesiology*, **78**, 1076–81.
Sartorelli, K. H., Abajian, J. C., Kreutz, J. M., and Vane, D. W. (1992). Improved outcome utilizing spinal anesthesia in high-risk infants. *Journal Pediatric Surgery*, **8**, 1022–5.
Watcha, M. F., Thach, B. T., and Gunter, J. B. (1989). Postoperative apnea after caudal anesthesia in an ex-premature infant. *Anesthesiology*, **71**, 613–15.
Welborn, L. G., Rice, L. J., Hannallah, R. S., Broadman, L. M., Ruttimann, U. E., and Fink, R. (1990). Postoperative apnea in former preterm infants: prospective comparison of spinal and general anesthesia. *Anesthesiology*, **72**, 838–42.

# SUBARACHNOID ANAESTHESIA IN AWAKE BABIES

## *Anatomy*

The spinal cord in a full-term baby extends to L3 and the dura to S3 or S4. The sacrum is not calcified until early adulthood. Lumbar puncture can be made below the termination of the spinal cord at the L4–L5, L5–S1 or S1–S2 interspaces. The pelvis in babies is proportionately smaller than in adults and the sacrum lies higher in relation to the iliac crests. The intercristal line indicates the position of L5–S1.

The depth of the subarachnoid space from the skin is approximately 7 mm in premature babies and 10 mm in full-term babies. A lumbar lordosis does not develop until about 12 months of age and this may alter the spread of local anaesthetics injected into the subarachnoid space.

The volume of cerebrospinal fluid in children less than 15 kg is 4 ml kg$^{-1}$, compared with 2 ml kg$^{-1}$ in adults, and it is equally divided between the brain and spine. The larger volume of cerebrospinal fluid may explain the relatively large volume of local anaesthetic needed for spinal anaesthesia in babies.

## *Indications*

Ex-premature babies having short operations on the lower abdomen or perineum including:

(1) circumcision;
(2) herniotomy;
(3) orchidopexy; and
(4) cystoscopy.

## *Contraindications*

(1) Local infection;
(2) septicaemia;
(3) coagulopathy;
(4) hydrocephalus;
(5) meningomyelocoele;
(6) local neurological disease;
(7) uncorrected hypotension.

## Equipment

### Needles

A needle used for subarachnoid anaesthesia in babies should have:

(1) a clear hub so that cerebrospinal fluid is easily seen;
(2) a stylet to reduce the risk of implantation dermoid;
(3) a short length so that it is easy to handle;
(4) a short bevel so that:
   (a) changes in tissue resistance are easily felt;
   (b) bone and cartilage are less easily penetrated;
   (c) the bevel is less likely to straddle the dura, leading to incomplete injection of local anaesthetic into the subarachnoid space,

The neonatal spinal needle (Becton and Dickinson UK Ltd) has these characteristics. It is 25 g and 2.5 cm long with a short bevel, a stylet, a clear hub and a needle dead-space of 0.05 ml. Atraumatic lumbar puncture needles are available but are neither ideal nor necessary:

(1) a 24 g 3.5 cm Sprotte needle is manufactured but the lateral aperture is 1.2 mm long. The aperture can straddle the dura, with the risk that only part of the dose of the local anaesthetic is injected into the subarachnoid space.
(2) a Whitacre needle has a lateral aperture lying immediately proximal to the pencil point, which is less likely to straddle the dura, but the needles are 9 cm long and are difficult to manipulate in babies.

### Syringes

A 1 ml syringe should be used because the volumes of local anaesthetic are very small.

### Filter needles

Local anaesthetic solutions should be drawn up through a filter needle to prevent injection of glass particles into the subarachnoid space.

### Drugs

Isobaric or hyperbaric solutions of bupivacaine 0.5 per cent in a dose according to weight (Table 14.1) with an allowance for the dead-space of the needle.

**Table 14.1**    Volume of (a) isobaric (Mahe and Ecoffey 1988) and (b) hyperbaric (Gallagher and Crean 1989) bupivacaine 0.5 per cent for subarachnoid anaesthesia in awake babies

| (a) | Body weight (kg) | Volume of bupivacaine (ml) |
|-----|------------------|----------------------------|
|     | < 2 | 0.25 |
|     | ≥ 2 but < 5 | 0.75 |
|     | ≥ 5 | 1.00 |
| (b) | $0.06 \text{ ml kg}^{-1} + 0.1 \text{ ml}$ | |

### Duration of action

Bupivacaine 0.5 per cent in a volume shown in Table 14.1(a) produces a motor block with a mean duration of 70 minutes (range: 20–110 minutes). Clinically, surgical anesthesia is unlikely to last more than 40 minutes. Adrenaline prolongs the duration of action of amethocaine (tetracaine) but not bupivacaine.

### Onset of block

Motor block usually occurs within 2–3 minutes.

### Success rate

Subarachnoid block is successful as the sole anaesthetic in about 90 per cent of ex-premature babies, although a second lumbar puncture may be needed to obtain an adequate height of block. Other local anaesthetic blocks (e.g. iliac crest block, infiltration with local anaesthetic of the wound, spermatic cord, or peritoneum) or sedation (inhalational or intravenous) are given to 5–10 per cent of babies because the height or duration of spinal block is inadequate. The most stimulating stages of inguinal herniotomy are deep dissection of the inguinal ring and traction on the spermatic cord or peritoneum. General anaesthesia is needed in a small number of babies, either because the subarachnoid space cannot be identified or the subsequent block is inadequate from the outset.

### Complications

The total experience of subarachnoid anaesthesia in babies is limited and there are few reports of serious complications. Complications reported include: a high block and postoperative apnoea. Potential complications include: neuropraxia, and haematoma.

## A high block

The height of block for a given volume of local anaesthetic varies from baby to baby, and a high block impairing the efficiency of breathing or causing apnoea can occasionally occur unpredictably.

A high block is more common in the following circumstances:

(1)  if a baby's legs are raised after subarachnoid block with hyperbaric solutions of local anaesthetics;

(2)  increasing the volume for a given concentration of local anaesthetic;

(3)  if caudal anaesthesia is used after failed subarachnoid block. It has been suggested that local anaesthetic may leak from the extradural to subarachnoid spaces through holes in the dura, but the reported complications may have occurred because of unrecognized puncture of the dura by the caudal needle.

The effect of the technique of injection (speed and barbotage) on the height of block in babies is unknown.

## Postoperative apnoea

The risk of apnoea after subarachnoid anaesthesia without sedation is probably decreased but not eliminated.

## Infection, haematoma, or neuropraxia.

These are potential complications not yet reported in babies.

## Difficulties

Technical problems account for most of the failures of spinal anaesthesia (Table 14.2).

## A 'dry tap'

Sometimes a definite 'pop' is felt, probably indicating puncture of the dura, but cerebrospinal fluid does not flow. A 'dry tap' may result from reduced hydrostatic pressure within the subarachnoid space, produced by dehydration or the baby lying in the lateral position. The needle should be gently aspirated with a 1 ml syringe. If cerebrospinal fluid still does not appear, lumbar puncture can be attempted with the baby in a sitting position.

**Table 14.2**  Failure rates and technical difficulties of subarachnoid anaesthesia among 142 ex-premature babies having minor surgery (herniotomy, circumcision, orchidopexy, or cystoscopy). Mean gestational age at birth 30.8 (SD 3.7) weeks; mean post-conceptual age at surgery 44.8 (SD 7.8) weeks; mean weight at surgery 3.3 (SD 1.2) kg (Sartorelli *et al.* 1992)

| Technical Difficulty | |
| --- | --- |
| Unable to obtain adequate anaesthesia before surgery | 4% |
| Second lumbar puncture needed | 26.8% |
| Inadequate anaesthesia during surgery | 6.3% |
| supplemented with: | |
| caudal block | 2 babies |
| nitrous oxide | 1 baby |
| intravenous sedation | 6 babies |

*A 'bloody tap'*

A 'bloody tap' is common in premature babies.

*Inadequate height or duration of block*

The height and duration of block is very variable between babies and the block cannot be extended. Some babies will need either a second lumbar puncture to obtain an adequate height of block. Occasionally a block that is satisfactory for the initial incision is inadequate during dissection of the deeper tissues of the abdominal wall or traction on the peritoneum or spermatic cord. Anaesthesia may be improved by other local anaesthetic techniques (e.g. iliac crest block, infiltration of the wound, hernial sac, or spermatic cord) or sedation (e.g. nitrous oxide, volatile agents, or intravenous drugs). A small number of babies will need general anaesthesia.

*Technique*

The electrocardiograph is monitored. The baby can be held in the left lateral position. The baby's hips are flexed but the head should be held slightly extended to prevent oxygen desaturation. The iliac crests and positions of the spines of L4, L5, and S1 are shown (Fig. 14.1).

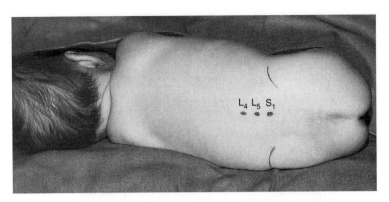

**Fig. 14.1**   The left lateral position for subarachnoid anaesthesia in babies. Both iliac crests and the spines of L4, L5, and S1 are marked.

Alternatively the baby can be held in the sitting position (Fig. 14.2). The greater hydrostatic pressure of the cerebrospinal fluid may reduce the chance of a 'dry tap'.

The lower back and buttocks are cleaned with an alcoholic antiseptic solution and draped with sterile towels. The point at which the needle is inserted is in the mid-line half way between the spinous processes of either L4–L5, L5–S1, or S1–S2, (Fig. 14.3). The skin is infiltrated with 1 per cent lignocaine using a 27 g needle, and a small nick is made with an 18 g needle. The lumbar puncture needle is then advanced at right-angles to the skin. The stylet should be removed frequently to look for cerebrospinal fluid. A 'pop' is sometimes felt as the dura is punctured. The depth of the subarachnoid space is about 7 mm in premature and 10 mm in full-term babies. Cerebrospinal fluid may not always flow because of the narrow bore of the needle or reduced hydrostatic pressure within the subarachnoid space. If cerebrospinal fluid does not appear, the needle should be gently aspirated with a syringe to confirm the position of the needle tip before local anaesthetic is injected.

The baby must be firmly held and the needle carefully stabilized as the syringe is attached and the local anaesthetic injected (Fig. 14.4). The needle tip is easily dislodged from the subarachnoid space with only small movements of the needle. Local anaesthetic is injected slowly over about 15–20 seconds without barbotage, and the needle is then removed. The baby is laid

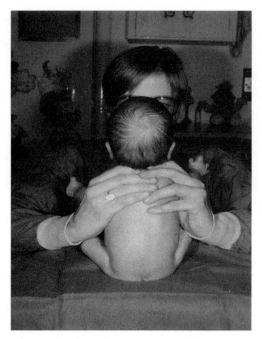

**Fig. 14.2**    The sitting position for subarachnoid anaesthesia in babies. The hips are flexed but the head is kept reasonably extended to prevent oxygen desaturation.

horizontally if isobaric solutions of local anaesthetic are used and slightly head-up if hyperbaric solutions are used. The block is usually established within 2–3 minutes.

## FURTHER READING

Yaster, M. and Maxwell, L. G. (1989). Pediatric regional anesthesia. *Anesthesiology*, **70**, 324–38.

## REFERENCES

Abajian, J. C., Mellish, R. W. P., Browne, A. F., Perkins, F. M., Lambert, D. H., and Mazuzan, J. E. (1984). Spinal anesthesia for surgery in the high-risk infant. *Anesthesia Analgesia*, **63**, 359–62.

Busoni, P. and Messeri, A. (1989). Spinal anaesthesia in children: surface anatomy. *Anesthesia Analgesia*, **68**, 413–23.

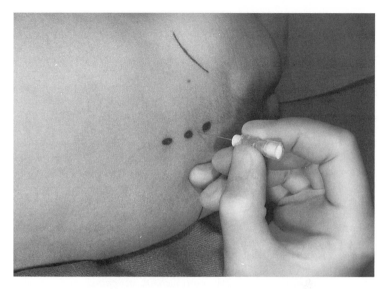

**Fig. 14.3**   Subarachnoid anaesthesia in babies. The needle is inserted midway between the spinous processes of L34, L45, L5, S1, or S2 at right angles to the skin.

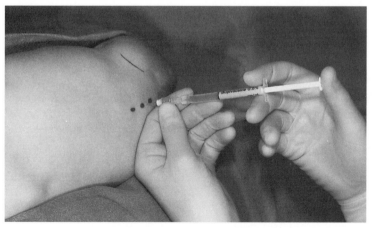

**Fig. 14.4**   A 1 ml syringe is used to inject local anaesthetics into the subarachnoid space. The baby must be firmly held and the needle carefully stabilized when attaching the syringe or injecting the local anaesthetic because the needle tip is easily displaced from the subarachnoid space.

Cox, R. G. and Goresky, G. V. (1990). Life-threatening apnea following spinal anesthesia in former premature infants. *Anesthesiology*, **73**, 345–7.

Desparmet, J. F. (1990). Total spinal anesthesia after caudal anesthesia in an infant. *Anesthesia Analgesia*, **70**, 665–7.

Gallagher, T. M. and Crean, P. M. (1989). Spinal anaesthesia in infants born prematurely. *Anaesthesia*, **44** , 434–6.

Gerber, A. C., Baitella, L. C., and Dangel, P. H. (1993). Spinal anaesthesia in former preterm infants. *Paediatric Anaesthesia*, **3**, 153–6.

Harnik, E. V., Hoy, G. R., Potolicchio, S., Stewart, D. R., and Siegelman, R. E. (1986). Spinal anesthesia in premature infants recovering from respiratory distress syndrome. *Anesthesiology*, **64**, 95–9.

Mahe, V. and Ecoffey, C. (1988). Spinal anesthesia with isobaric bupivacaine in infants. *Anesthesiology*, **68**, 601–3.

Sartorelli, K. H., Abajian, J. C., Kreutz, J. M., and Vane, D. W. (1992). Improved outcome utilizing spinal anesthesia in high-risk infants. *Journal Pediatric Surgery*, **27**, 1022–5.

Welborn, L. G., Rice, L. J., Hannallah, R. S., Broadman, L. M., Ruttimann, U. E., and Fink, R. (1990). Postoperative apnea in former preterm infants: prospective comparison of spinal and general anesthesia. *Anesthesiology*, **72**, 838–42.

Wright, T. E., Orr, R. J., Haberkern, C. M., and Walbergh, E. J. (1990). Complications during spinal anesthesia in infants: high spinal blockade. *Anesthesiology*, **73**, 1290–2.

# CAUDAL EXTRADURAL ANAESTHESIA IN AWAKE BABIES

### Anatomy

The sacral hiatus lies at the apex of an equilateral triangle formed by the posterior superior iliac spines. It is covered by the sacrococcygeal membrane and forms a shallow depression between the sacral cornua above the sacrococcygeal joint.

The sacrum in a baby is cartilaginous and relatively flat compared with older children and adults. The dura extends as far as S3 or S4.

(See also pp. 202–15.)

### Indications

Ex-premature babies having short operations on the lower abdomen or perineum, including:

(1) circumcision;
(2) herniotomy;
(3) orchidopexy; and
(4) cystoscopy.

## Contraindications

(1) Local sepsis;
(2) septicaemia;
(3) coagulopathy;
(4) local neurological disease;
(5) meningomyelocoele;
(6) hydrocephalus;
(7) uncorrected hypotension;
(8) major malformations of the sacrum.

## Equipment

### Needles

A 20 g intravenous cannula (e.g. Abbocath-T® Abbot Laboratories), is ideal for caudal extradural anaesthesia in awake babies, because:

(1) the needle functions as a stylet, reducing the risk of an implantation dermoid;
(2) there is a very positive 'feel' as the shoulders of the cannula penetrate the sacro-coccygeal membrane;
(3) the cannula can be advanced 1–1.5 cm over the needle and is less likely to become dislodged if the baby moves;
(4) epidural catheters can be threaded through the cannula.

### Filter needles

Local anaesthetic should be drawn up through a filter needle or injected through a filter to exclude particles of glass.

### Drugs

*Single injection of local anaesthetic through a cannula*
Bupivacaine 0.25 per cent 1 ml kg$^{-1}$.

*Local anaesthetic injected through a caudal catheter*
Initial injection of bupivacaine 0.25 per cent 0.7 ml kg$^{-1}$ and subsequent injections of bupivacaine 0.25 per cent 0.3 ml kg$^{-1}$

40 minutes after the first dose or earlier if clinically indicated (maximum of 1 ml kg$^{-1}$ in the first hour).

### Duration of action

The duration of anaesthesia produced by the first dose of local anaesthetic is approximately 45 minutes.

### Onset of block

10–15 minutes.

### Complications

#### Subarachnoid injection of local anaesthetic

Injection of local anaesthetic into the subarachnoid space will produce a 'total spinal block'. Dural puncture is more likely if:

(1)  the dura extends to a lower level than normal;
(2)  the laminae of other sacral vertebrae are not fused, so that the needle can be inadvertently inserted into the sacral canal at a higher segmental level;
(3)  the caudal needle is inserted more than a few millimetres into the sacral canal.

The clinical features of a 'total spinal' block in a baby include:

(1)  ventilatory arrest;
(2)  loss of consciousness;
(3)  dilated pupils.

Hypotension is not usually a feature. Ventilation must be supported but surgery can continue if the baby is haemodynamically stable. The block resolves within 1–2 hours.

#### Intravascular or intraosseous injection of local anaesthetic

Intravascular or intraosseous injection of local anaesthetic may produce convulsions or cardiac toxicity (see p. 208).

#### Penetration of the sacrum

Penetration of the sacrum by the needle may damage pelvic viscera or blood vessels.

*Postoperative apnoea*

The incidence of apnoea is probably reduced, *but not eliminated*, by caudal block compared with general anaesthesia.

*Haematoma and abscess formation*

These potential complications have not been reported in babies.

*Technique*

An intravenous cannula is inserted and the electrocardiograph monitored. The baby is held securely over the shoulder of an assistant, with the legs bent (Fig. 14.5), or firmly in the lateral position with the hips flexed but the head reasonably extended to prevent oxygen desaturation (Fig. 14.6). The skin over the lower back and buttocks is cleaned with an alcoholic antiseptic solution and draped with sterile towels. The sacral hiatus is found either:

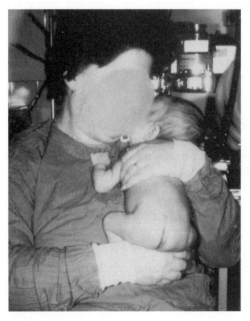

**Fig. 14.5**   The baby can be held securely over the shoulder of an assistant during caudal injection.

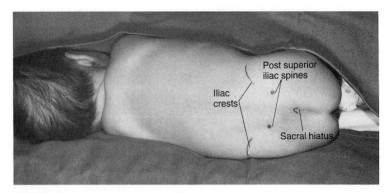

**Fig. 14.6** Left lateral position and the landmarks for caudal anaesthesia in a baby.

(1) as a shallow depression at the apex of an equilateral triangle formed by the posterior superior iliac spines and in the midline, or

(2) at the end of a line running along the lateral border of the uppermost thigh.

This skin over the sacral hiatus is infiltrated with 1 per cent lignocaine using a 27 g needle.

The caudal needle should be inserted between the sacral cornua and advanced in a sagittal plane at an angle of about 15° to the skin (Fig. 14.7). A 'pop' is felt as the shoulders of the cannula penetrate the sacro-coccygeal membrane. The sacro-coccygeal membrane is within a few millimetres of the skin.

The intravenous cannula is advanced 2–3 mm and then held securely as the cannula is advanced 1–1.5 cm over the needle stylet (Fig. 14.8). The needle stylet is then removed. After gentle aspiration with a syringe, local anaesthetic is injected slowly. A sensory block develops over about 15 minutes. The height of block is assessed before surgery by pinching the skin over the site of incision.

Extradural catheters can be inserted in awake babies (Fig. 14.9) (see pp. 215–22). For inguinal herniotomy the tip of the catheter should be advanced only about 5 cm so that local anaesthetic produces both a sensory block within the operative field and weakness of the legs. Increments of local anaesthetic can be given to extend the height or duration of block.

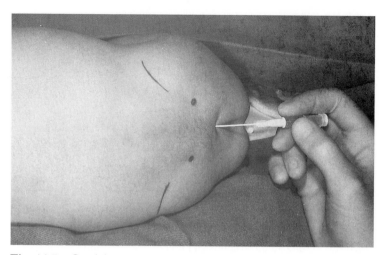

**Fig. 14.7**    Caudal anaesthesia in a baby. The caudal needle or cannula should be inserted between the sacral cornua and advanced in a saggital plane at an angle of about 15° to the skin.

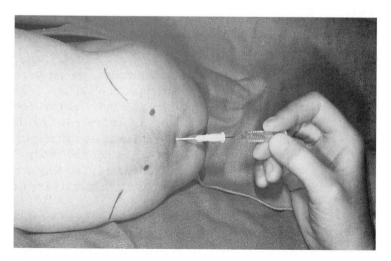

**Fig. 14.8**    If an intravenous cannula is used, the cannula can be advanced 1–1.5 cm over the needle once the sacro-coccygeal membrane is penetrated.

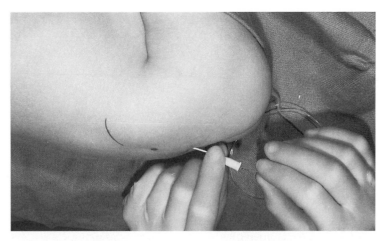

**Fig. 14.9** Using an intravenous cannula to site extradural catheters from the sacral hiatus in a baby.

## REFERENCES

Gunter, J. B., *et al.* (1991). Caudal epidural anesthesia in conscious premature and high-risk infants. *Journal of Pediatric Surgery*, **26**, 9–14.

Peutrell, J. M. and Hughes, D. G. (1993). Epidural anaesthesia through caudal catheters for inguinal herniotomies in awake ex-premature babies. *Anaesthesia*, **47**, 128–31.

Spear, R. M., Deshpande, J. K., and Maxwell, L. G. (1988). Caudal anesthesia in the awake, high-risk infant. *Anesthesiology*, **69**, 407–9.

# Index